Keith Cox is a highly qualified nurse who has dedicated 50 years of his life to patient care, mentoring cancer nurses, writing research papers and addressing medical conferences around the world. In 2006, he was the third-ever Australian to become a cancer nurse practitioner and in 2007 he was awarded an OAM for his services to nursing and community volunteer work. Keith remains involved with various fundraising committees and charitable organisations, and he volunteers in several capacities.

Grant Jones is a former newspaper and radio journalist, editor and TV researcher and producer, with more than three decades' experience. He now runs his own media consultancy business. Grant lives in Drummoyne with his partner, Joan, and their teenage son, Louis. Grant joins Keith, who lives a few blocks away, at their local gym three times a week. This is his first book.

T0283089

A CARING LIFE

KEITH COX
WITH GRANT JONES

MACMILLAN
Pan Macmillan Australia

Pan Macmillan acknowledges the Traditional Custodians of country throughout Australia and their connections to lands, waters and communities. We pay our respect to Elders past and present and extend that respect to all Aboriginal and Torres Strait Islander peoples today. We honour more than sixty thousand years of storytelling, art and culture.

Some of the people in this book have had their names changed to protect their identities.

First published 2022 in Macmillan by Pan Macmillan Australia Pty Ltd
1 Market Street, Sydney, New South Wales, Australia, 2000

Copyright © Keith Cox and Grant Jones 2022

The moral right of the authors to be identified as the authors of this work has been asserted.

All rights reserved. No part of this book may be reproduced or transmitted by any person or entity (including Google, Amazon or similar organisations), in any form or by any means, electronic or mechanical, including photocopying, recording, scanning or by any information storage and retrieval system, without prior permission in writing from the publisher.

A catalogue record for this book is available from the National Library of Australia

Typeset in Bembo by Midland Typesetters, Australia
Printed by IVE

Excerpt on pages 57–58 courtesy of *Canberra Times*/ACM.
Extract on page 200 from *I Am Gail* by Juliette O'Brien,
HarperCollins Publishers Australia Pty Limited.
Excerpt on page 224 from 'Cannonball', Words and Music by Damien Rice, © 2003
Warner/Chappell Music, Ltd. All Rights Reserved. Used by Permission of Alfred Music.

Any health or medical content contained in this book is not intended as health or medical advice. The publishers and their respective employees, agents and authors are not liable for injuries or damage occasioned to any person as a result of reading or following any health or medical content contained in this book.

The author and the publisher have made every effort to contact copyright holders for material used in this book. Any person or organisation that may have been overlooked should contact the publisher.

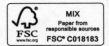

The paper in this book is FSC® certified. FSC® promotes environmentally responsible, socially beneficial and economically viable management of the world's forests.

This book is dedicated to the medical professionals who devote their lives to others, and to the families of those who have lost loved ones to cancer.

CONTENTS

'It must never be lost sight of what observation is for. It is not for the sake of piling up miscellaneous information or curious facts, but for the sake of saving life and increasing health and comfort.'

– Florence Nightingale (1859)

FOREWORD

When Keith and I first met in 1981, I was in my third year of medical school, which is the first time you see patients as a student training to be a doctor. By the early 1990s, when I began working as an oncologist, the causes of many cancers had been identified. However, cancer treatment then was still quite crude by today's standards. It was already clear that to treat cancer effectively an entire team was required, with physiotherapists and psychologists and, of course, highly competent and supportive nurses. Keith also knew that and that's how we started working together. He was one of those people who already understood the importance of teamwork and most important of all, the support patients needed, both emotional and physical, to get them through their cancer treatment.

It wasn't an accident either that there were similarities in the way we both wanted to treat patients, as we both knew treatment is driven by what you see and what you think is needed.

Neither of us were satisfied with maintaining the status quo. If we thought there was a better way to do things, then we would work together on how we could do that and then implement change.

By the late 1980s, Keith had gained another reputation because he and a coterie of chemotherapy nurses dubbed 'KC and the Sunshine Band' and later known as 'Keith and the Chemettes' would parade through the wards administering cancer treatment. While Keith had a reputation for organising the serious stuff, such as cancer treatment, he was also renowned for organising all the parties and making the fun stuff happen as well, like car rallies and cocktail parties and cake-making competitions.

By 2006, much later in our careers, he asked me to help him be recognised as a nurse practitioner, which I thought was a fabulous idea. He knew that if he was able to do more of the things that needed doing, such as the prescribing and administering of cancer drug treatments, without having to wait for someone else – including a doctor – to come and do it, that our patients would benefit. To me, this is where the field of cancer treatment needed to go, so I fully endorsed it. To provide the very best care, specialist nurses with great expertise who know how to treat people are a key requirement.

When I took over from Professor Chris O'Brien as Director of the Sydney Cancer Centre that same year, after Chris was diagnosed with brain cancer, Keith and I had very similar ideas about how we could execute his vision for a new state-of-the-art cancer treatment centre. A year after Chris died, the old Page Chest Pavilion at Royal Prince Alfred Hospital (RPA) was pulled down and Lifehouse was built. After it was completed, I thought: 'This is stuff that we had all talked about – Chris, Keith and I – all these ideas that we had worked on for many, many years are now a reality.'

At the time, Keith was one of just three cancer nurse practitioners in Australia, so he's always been a bit of a ground-breaker and a pioneer for the cancer cause. Keith is also technically highly skilled and a competent nurse and I think you have to go a very, very long way to find a person with more compassion and care. The same compassion and care that he shows for patients, he also shows for colleagues. Plus he sets a very high standard of quality so it's like he has all the good bits of being a perfectionist and none of the bad. That is one of his very good traits because, in health care, you want to get it right. If you don't get it right, bad things happen to people.

Keith has also long realised that there is always a better way to look after patients. His passion for nursing goes way beyond normal patient care. It's more than just feeling sorry for someone, though: it's understanding what they are going through and knowing intuitively what he – both as a nurse and a human being – needs to do to help them through it. He doesn't feel like it's his job or his duty either. He feels that it's a privilege.

There would not have been too many days between 1993 (when I returned to RPA from overseas) and when Keith retired in 2018 that we haven't spoken about a patient or I hadn't called him for advice. I know a lot of things but I don't know everything, and there's a bunch of things that he has in that vast bank of knowledge that I can tap into. While there are now other cancer nurse practitioners, it's hard to find someone with 40 years of experience and who just has it in their bones, if you like. Someone who just *gets it*!

– Michael Boyer AM
Chief Clinical Officer, Chris O'Brien Lifehouse

1

NOT THE FIRST, NOT THE LAST

While I have travelled the world, lived overseas, met a future king, greeted premiers, consoled a prime minister, stood side by side with medical pioneers and met other famous people, I will always be a humble country boy at heart. My parents, Bill and Pansy Cox, married in the St Francis Xavier Catholic Church in Gunning, New South Wales, in 1934. Dad was a cabinet-maker by trade and grew up in Sydney, in St Peters. Mum, meanwhile, was from a farming family and her dad managed Boorowa, a property on the Southern Tablelands of NSW, while she worked as a cook and governess. Dad moved to the area and turned his trade to building houses, and later built St Silas's Anglican Church, which still stands on the fringes of the bleached-blond hayfields of the Breadalbane Plain. After they met, fell in love and married, the young couple, with two kids in tow, bought a two-bedroom railway fettlers' cottage at Cullerin, then a speck of a town between Goulburn and Gunning. This is where I was born.

They named their new home 'FayBri' after their first-born girl, Fay, and first-born boy, Brian, but many more children were to come. After Fay was Coral, Dawn, then Brian, Ronnie and Judy. Mum had me when she was 38, Loretta at 41, and baby Vincent came along when Mum was 44. In the end, of the nine Cox children, only six of us were ever living at home at any one time because, as each new child was born, one of the older chickadees – as Mum called us – was ready to fly the nest.

I fondly recall that nest in Cullerin as a large house with many rooms, which Dad was constantly adding to. Our patch sat below the verge of a hill, in a dip just after the railway crossing. The cottage was on the edge of a thin ribbon of land sandwiched between the old Hume Highway and the main 630-mile train line connecting Sydney and Melbourne. The road was a treacherous stretch of tar which was then well known as the deadliest in the state, and the railway line seemed so close that I'd swear the Spirit of Progress was passing straight through my bedroom, leaving a plume of diesel smoke on its way to Albury.

Mum and Dad ran the general store and we also had a cow, several orphaned lambs, sometimes pigs, and an egg farm supplied by a thousand chooks. One of my early jobs was cleaning out the chook sheds, not a fun thing to do, especially as I had asthma. On the rare occasion when Mum was away, we'd ask, 'What are we having for tea, Dad?' and inevitably the answer would be, 'What about eggs? I have plenty of cracked ones.' To this day, eggs are not my favourite food. There was a shed for our milking cow, at one stage some pigpens, and the chook sheds were right next to the road. We also had a small orchard, a veggie garden tucked up beside a lane which led to the railway line, and a little paddock for the orphaned sheep.

It was a dry and sparse landscape so in addition to the rainwater tank by the house, we ran water for the septic tank and the livestock, including our chooks, from a dam.

As an ever-increasing number of cars and trucks started making their way up and down the Hume Highway, my enterprising dad poured a concrete apron on the crest of the hill and installed a couple of petrol bowsers. After refuelling, customers would walk down the incline to our little general store, which sold necessary supplies such as cereal, milk, eggs from our chooks, bread, tinned goods, cigarettes and milkshakes. There was also plenty of oil and fan belts and the like for motorists. It was a pickup point for mail, and served as the local telephone exchange as well. We almost backed onto Cullerin railway station and its canvas tent village which was home to the railway fettlers who, more often than not, were migrant workers. They'd come into the shop and Mum would announce the names of the dry goods or produce as they pointed. 'Sugar', 'tea', 'potatoes', 'biscuits', 'bread', she'd say.

We also had fresh milk from our cow and we kids would fight over scooping the cream off the top of the billy can. More often than not, the second-in-line Coral – my eldest sister, Fay, had already left home by then – used to win the fight for the cream. I can't remember if everyone liked the cream – I know I did – but the rest of us would spread what remained of it on a slice of bread topped with strawberry jam. If there was ever any left over, Mum would hand-beat it with a mixer, turning it into butter. By the time baby Vincent arrived on the scene, we no longer had a milking cow. Instead, Dad would pick up the milk in big stainless-steel milk cans from Dairy Farmers in Goulburn, once a week, and take them back to the shop where customers would fill up their own glass milk bottles with a ladle. In later years, it would be crates of bottled milk.

As our family grew, Dad, the carpenter and cabinet-maker, was constantly adding to our cottage. To keep us occupied, he also built a merry-go-round, see-saw, monkey bars, two swings, a trapeze swing and an igloo-shaped cubby house which had a concrete floor. While we didn't have a need to go anywhere, we did anyway. It was mostly exploring at 'the crevices', a series of earthen corridors eroded over time by a small creek, or to our neighbours' places, a few hundred yards away, to ride their horses. Just up the hill was our primary school, which we attended with the many children from other families who lived nearby. Dad started to dig a hole for a swimming pool, too, but sadly it remained a mere hole in the ground until my elderly parents left the property several decades later. Dad levelled a piece of ground for a tennis court as well, but that also remained unfinished, as did a proposed master bedroom for my parents that never got further than a set of footings and a single wall.

Despite being incomplete, our Cullerin home was full of love and care and a place where we enjoyed growing up, exploring and working as a big family. I only realise today how hard Mum and Dad must have worked. Dad would get up at dawn to unlock the petrol bowsers and take the oil out of the shed; he'd feed the chooks, gather and pack eggs and open the shop. Meanwhile, Mum would wrangle the children, getting us younger kids off to primary school or the older ones on the bus to high school in Gunning. Then she would run the shop, post office and telephone exchange in between juggling all the domestic chores, including the washing on a Monday. All our clothes and the linen were boiled up in the copper, then put through the handwringer before being hung up on the line and wherever else she could find room. In winters, back then, there was occasionally enough snow to close the roads, which meant the bus couldn't get the older ones to high school. But Dad and Mum always had things for us to do, so they'd enjoy those few extra hands around the house for a day or two.

On my recent return, the reality of the property was different from my fond memories. The farm must have been a lot smaller than I recall, tiny in fact, and probably is what we'd now recognise as a hobby farm. But it was a happy place to grow up.

2

A DING-DONG BREAK-IN AT CULLERIN

My parents always thought I was a bit of a stickybeak so our shop, post office and petrol station proved an ideal spot for me to sit, watch and generally hang around. These were the days when the business was quite busy, as we were the only store for miles and there was nothing like a supermarket in existence. Our customers were mostly locals who came in from their farms to pick up groceries, grab their mail, top up with petrol or just have a chat – although usually all four. Everyone around knew us and we knew them, but, of course, there was also a stream of strangers making their way up and down the highway, as well as a local truck driver or two.

When I wasn't at school or helping out on the farm, I used to love sitting in the shop, listening to the various conversations and watching all the comings and goings. In a way, I suppose, watching those people was an early indication of my inquisitive nature and probably the reason why I still ask so many questions today. It's possibly also the reason I remember so clearly the incident that happened in the summer holidays of 1962. I was 12, so I had plenty of time after chores on the farm to see all the things that were happening around me. As usual, Mum was serving in the shop when two men walked in and started asking all these strange questions: 'What time do you close?', 'Who else is here?', 'What else do you sell?' and other queries which just sounded odd coming from two strangers.

Later that night we were all in bed, sound asleep, when my mother heard the shop doorbell. On hot summer days, we always left the main door with the brass bell open during business hours, only using the screen door – and that didn't have a bell on it. As the brass bell was attached to the main entry door – which Dad had recently renovated – when you entered it went 'ding', and when the door closed behind you, it went 'dong'. How many thousands of times had I heard that bell? I don't know, but obviously whoever was breaking into our shop in the dead of night didn't know the bell was there. My father was always late going to bed and hardly ever ate dinner with us because he'd either be in the fowl sheds, rolling the oil stands away into the garage, locking up the bowsers or adding up the ledgers at the close of business. After a late dinner, he was usually exhausted, so was a sound sleeper. He didn't hear a thing.

It was probably one o'clock in the morning when the doorbell woke Mum. On her side of the bed, there was a door that led to the bathroom but the main door to the hall was on my father's side of the bed. So she jumped over Dad and started creeping up the hall. She suddenly heard a knock and shouted, 'Who's there?' Well, everyone in the house was awake by this time, including my older brothers Brian and Ronnie, 20 and 18 by then, who shared a room just off the hall. With Mum singing out and flicking on all the light switches, the boys jumped out of bed and joined her in the hall. With that, they all heard the 'dong' of the door closing, but by the time they got to the shop, no one was there. We had a big driveway that came up alongside the store, while the petrol bowsers were up nearer the highway, so the boys turned off all our shop lights to try to spot a retreating car in the dark. As there was no sign of car lights outside, they agreed that whoever it was who was trying to get in was on foot and decided to jump into Brian's car and head towards Goulburn to see if they could track them down.

My brothers drove up to a place called Mutmutbilly Creek. They parked the car on the hill and turned off the headlights. Two fellows soon emerged from the darkness, walking along the road, a couple of hundred yards away. They must have ducked off when they saw the boys' headlights coming their way, then waited for the car to pass. Instead, Brian and Ronnie were waiting for them at the crest of the hill and aimed to jump out and grab the fugitives when they passed. But before the pair got to the car, they disappeared again into the paddocks and my brothers couldn't find them anywhere. After a fruitless search in the dark, they came home empty-handed.

Dad was well awake by then and had surveyed the scene, devastated most of all by the damage that had been done to his new door. Applying his talent as a carpenter, Dad had just finished renovating the whole shop, and the main entry was his pride and joy. The refurbishments had included a new timber and plate glass door with a shiny chrome handle and nice wooden trim at the bottom. While Dad saw the timber trim as a highlight, the thieves saw it as a weak point and had used an old-fashioned brace and bit to drill several holes in the bottom. It appeared they'd wanted to weaken the trim sufficiently so that they could punch through a bigger hole and one of them could wriggle inside and gain access to all the goodies in our shop.

They hadn't really thought this through, however. We had one of those red telephone boxes out the front, on the left of the driveway, and when we discovered the brace and bit they'd used outside it, we worked out what had happened. Every time a car or semitrailer had zoomed past on the highway, it would have lit up their location at the front doorstep, so the thieves must have been running back and forth to the telephone box to hide. As well as that, they would have been unable to rotate their old-fashioned drill efficiently, as it would have kept hitting the front step. At some point they must have had enough, and turned their attention elsewhere. While our shopfront consisted of fixed plate glass windows and Dad's new door, above one window were some louvres.

'Here's a better idea!' one of these geniuses must have said to his mate. 'You give me a leg up and I'll take the louvres out of the top window.'

So one aspiring thief took out the louvres one at a time, handing them down to his mate who ran behind the phone box and dropped them there. Then one thief boosted the other up through the gap. After he dropped down into the shop, he went to open the door to let his mate in, which is when the doorbell dinged. The thieves probably realised too late that when the door closed behind them a 'dong' would follow. It was the early '60s, we were in the country, and you left your car unlocked in those days. Sometimes you even left the keys in it, so security was light to say the least, but all it took was a simple brass bell to signal the alarm. And when these two ding-dongs had cased the joint earlier in the day, they hadn't realised they'd make a racket when they opened the main shop door.

Mum had already phoned the police but as there was no station in Cullerin, the police would have to come from further away in Goulburn or Gunning. When they did eventually arrive, in the early hours of the morning, there was a great deal of excitement and the whole household was awake, the six of us kids who were still at home, my parents and two Gunning policemen all gathered around the kitchen table. The police took statements and with me being the stickybeak that I was, I gave them a fairly good description of the cagey pair who had entered our shop earlier that day.

'I'm sure it was those fellows. They were very suspicious,' Mum said. She was convinced they were a couple of railway fettlers. No doubt she would have been filling the kettle and putting on a calming cup of tea as she voiced her suspicions, and offering her famous sponge cake as well. Meanwhile, given that the thieves had fled empty-handed, Dad's biggest concern was all the damage that had been done to his new door.

As is the way in small country towns, by morning the whole of Cullerin and the surrounding district knew we'd had a break-in. Our neighbour Paul Hannan, who owned the property around where the fellows had disappeared into the night, told police he'd seen someone at Mutmutbilly Creek early that morning. There were two old stone walls still standing sentinel from an 1800s settlers' house and Paul felt the pair must have camped out behind them for the night before moving on the following morning. Country people always start work early, heading out into the paddocks just before dawn and doing a couple of hours work before breakfast, so Paul must have called the police bright and early.

'I think I've spotted the two guys who broke into the Coxes',' he said. 'They've headed towards the road near the Breadalbane Plains.'

The Goulburn police called their colleagues at Collector, a town 20 miles away. We later heard the Collector police were driving along the road, just past the Breadalbane Plains, when they spotted two men trying to hitch a ride. 'Would you like a lift, gentlemen? Hop in!' one officer said as they pulled alongside. 'We've also got a few questions for you,' he added as the pair reluctantly got into the police car.

So a lift to the police station ended up with a stay in the cells until the alleged thieves' court appearance before the local magistrate the next morning. After giving my statement, I was excited to think I might be heading to the beautiful 1880s Goulburn Court House in Montague Street to identify the culprits. But when they appeared before the magistrate, I wasn't called to give evidence and they were convicted as charged. The duo appealed and the case went to the District Court, in Darlinghurst, Sydney. This is where I thought I'd get my chance. The witnesses, Dad, Ronnie, Brian and myself, all left for Sydney to give evidence, leaving my poor mum at home to look after the chooks, the post office, shop, petrol bowsers and the rest of the kids.

My father's mother was still alive then and had a house in St Peters, right on the Princes Highway, opposite the old brickworks, so we stayed with her instead of using the small amount of money for accommodation and food given to us by the court. Grandma's was a dark three-bedroom house, filled wall-to-wall with my own dad's oil paintings – he had been an amateur painter in his younger days. I was given a little room to myself and spent that afternoon exploring her courtyard, which included a little fishpond and a mosaic of collected seashells cemented to the walls of a small garden bed. Both the coal man and the ice man arrived that day to make their deliveries, all of which was a big event for a young boy from Cullerin who was a long way from home. The next day, we headed off to Darlinghurst Court and sat in a big waiting room in our Sunday best, all excited and ready to give evidence. My father went in first, then my brothers one by one, then our neighbour Paul Hannan. I was going to be the last to give my side of the story but just before I was to head in, the prosecutor came into the room. 'We don't need you. The judge has enough to convict.'

So the biggest day of my then 12-year life turned out to be a big disappointment, but we did receive a paid trip to Sydney and got to visit my grandma. While we were supposed to stay for two nights, we only stayed one as the court case was over so quickly and Dad was keen to get back home. It also meant we could save a bit of money. Later, after all the fuss, the convicted pair appealed again, and while I didn't have to come back to court for their third appearance, Dad did, and he complained about it dragging on for such a long time.

'That bloody old judge,' said my father on his return. 'I'm sure he had diarrhoea because he kept adjourning the court and going out and coming back in half an hour later. Then he couldn't remember what had been said before.'

The pair were eventually acquitted on their third appearance, but in the meantime had spent quite a bit of time in Goulburn

Gaol and at Darlinghurst Court lock-up, so they didn't get away scot-free. Weeks later, Dad received an anonymous letter at our Cullerin post office: *Borers in your door, silverfish galore! Get a Flick man, that's your answer, remember one Flick, and they're gone!* which was a nod to a well-known TV and radio jingle at the time, and now to Dad's holey door. The letter wasn't signed, but Dad knew exactly who it was from.

As for the money from my court appearance, like most kids back then, my parents had started a school account for me. Mondays were bank days, and at the start of every school week, all us school kids were given two shillings to put in our Commonwealth Bank account. The money for my non-existent court appearance went into that. I can't remember how much it was but at the time it seemed like a fortune. So crime did pay, at least for me.

Two decades later, the excitement of that break-in turned to tragedy as my parents faced another burglary, this time a serious one that would result in a violent home invasion and an assault that left a crippling legacy. The year after the thwarted robbery, I headed off to Gunning to the combined primary and high school.

3

SISTER FAY – THE FLY-IN NUN

In her own teenage years, my sister Fay, the eldest of the Cox children, put a lot of faith in God. She left school around 15 to head to St John of God Hospital in Goulburn to train as a nurse, but her real aspiration was to become a nun. The St John of God order was started by pioneering Catholic Sisters from Ireland who had devoted their lives in service to the sick. The order had eventually built hospitals throughout Australia, with patients cared for by the nuns in their big white wimples who had also trained as nurses. But as there was no nursing training in Goulburn, Fay worked at St John of God Hospital as an assistant nurse.

When Fay was told by Mum and Dad that we were expecting a new arrival in several months time, she vowed that if our new sibling was a girl, it was the Lord telling her to join the convent, but if it was a boy, then God was telling Fay to remain with the family. Three months after our youngest sister, Loretta, was born, Fay, aged 17, boarded a train in Goulburn with our parents' blessing and arrived in Perth three days later. Soon after that, she landed at St John of God Convent in Subiaco where she would become a novice nun. At the age of 21, Fay Eunice Cox would take her final vows and be given another name, Sister Chrysostom, after John Chrysostom (347–407 CE), a scholar and author who later became Archbishop of Constantinople. Coral, who by then was 20 and a trainee nurse at St John of God Hospital, and the next sibling down in the pecking order, was the only member of the family to board the train to Perth to attend Fay's final profession. As Fay was 14 when I came along and I was three when she left home, I didn't remember much about her at all and we wouldn't see her again for another 13 years.

To us younger ones, our only understanding of Fay's life as a nurse and nun was through the frequent letters she wrote to Mum, who would read them out loud to us. Every Saturday morning, Mum used to take all the furniture out of the breakfast room and kitchen before dropping down on her hands and knees to scrub the floors. Off the breakfast room was the courtyard and off that was the laundry, so everything was bundled outside to give Mum a clear space to wash the floors properly. After checking the mail, dropped off by the morning train, Mum would call us all in from the paddocks and yards. 'We've got a letter from Fay,' she'd say. Occasionally, accompanying the letter would be a photo of Sister Chrys in the stiff wimple of the nun's habit, and we would look upon this vision in white with wonder. Letters were the only communication we had with Sister Chrys for about a decade and while we had a telephone, calls were rare, very expensive and a luxury the nuns avoided.

It was with great joy one Saturday that Mum announced that Fay was coming home to visit. Mum was beside herself with excitement, of course, so the floors were never finished that morning and the chairs and table remained outside as we all absorbed the news. In hindsight, it was like we were told royalty was coming to visit, and it felt like preparations for her arrival went on for months. While there was much anticipation about Fay's trip and my parents went to extremes to make everything nice, just before Fay was due home, Mum started to get anxious. 'She's not going to be able to stay here because she's a nun,' she'd tell us. 'She'll have to stay in Goulburn at St John's Hospital.' Mum presumed this was the case because that's where Fay had been nursing before entering the convent in Perth. 'We won't get to see her,' she'd tell Dad. In addition, the very busy business of running the poultry farm and looking after the other animals was never-ending, so Mum thought we wouldn't be able to go into Goulburn to visit Fay at the convent. Mum wrote back:

It's lovely that you are coming home, dear, but it's going to be quite hard because of the business, so how often are we going to see you?

I don't need to stay in Goulburn, Mum, I can stay at home, Fay replied. So there was relief and great excitement once again in the Cox household. But Mum had more doubts. 'How are we going to get her to Mass every day?' she asked Dad. There was only a little stone church nearby, St Brigid's at Breadalbane where I was baptised, but it didn't have a daily Mass. And it couldn't be St Silas's, the church that Dad built, as that was Anglican, and besides, it didn't have a daily service either. But there was the grand church in Goulburn, St Peter and Paul's Old Cathedral, which Mum deemed good enough for Fay to say her prayers. The journey to Goulburn was considered a long way back then and Mum didn't drive. My two elder brothers, who did, worked, and Dad was needed at the petrol station, shop and farm. How would Fay get into town to say her daily Mass and her Divine Office – the prayers all priests and nuns say morning and night? Fay would be stranded, churchless in Cullerin!

Fay wrote back: *I don't need to go to Mass every day, Mum, as long as I can go on Sundays and I'll just say extra prayers and the Divine Office.*

So that was that! Fay was coming home, she could pray and go to Mass, but as there were still six of us kids living at home, we had to find somewhere for her to sleep.

'We'll put her in the billiard room,' Dad said. 'I'll paint it, too.' He also ordered new linen and a new eiderdown as, by the time Fay was due to arrive home, it would be the middle of winter and very cold, especially compared to Perth.

Mum didn't go to Sydney to meet Fay on the day she was due to fly in, leaving it to the eldest boy Brian and his new fiancée, Joyce. They drove from Cullerin to the airport at Mascot and picked up Fay after the Perth flight touched down at about seven o'clock that night. With the return trip from Sydney to Cullerin taking about four hours, and a pit stop at Coral's place in Moss Vale scheduled on the way through, it would be a very late royal arrival.

'You kids go to bed and I'll wake you at about a quarter to midnight. They should be here around then,' Mum said as she fussed about the house. Mum also announced that we would be having a midnight tea in the lounge room, normally reserved for special guests. There was a window at the end of the room where the formal dining table and chairs overlooked Dad's concrete fishpond. At the other end was the lounge and off this room was the billiard room/aka Fay's bedroom. In the lounge room, opposite Fay's room, were a set of French doors that led to my narrow room which was just wide enough to fit a single bed. Dad was still finishing off painting the billiard room as we went to bed late that night, while Mum made Fay's bed ready for her arrival in the early hours. Bill and Pansy Cox were exhausted but the happiest they'd been for a long time knowing that their eldest daughter, who they hadn't seen for 13 years, would soon be home. As I drifted off to sleep to the lingering smell of fresh paint, I wondered what Fay was going to be like.

'Up you get,' Mum said as she woke us. 'They'll all be here soon and I've got the fire on in the lounge room so it will be nice and warm for you all.'

She put the kettle on for tea to accompany the fresh sponge cake and biscuits she had made and it wasn't long before our royal guest arrived via the shop door. As you may recall, our shopfront had two doors, one main door with a big plate glass window in it, plus a screen door to keep the flies out. So here was our special visitor, dressed in a simple black nun's habit, on the inside of the screen door but on the outside of the main door, with my excited mother looking at her through the glass. Mum pulled one way but Fay was pulling the other way as all of us sleepy-eyed kids stood there gawking. Outside, Brian brushed past his big sister and said, 'Look, let me do it, Fay,' and pushed open the door. So, after more than a decade – and a few seconds while they struggled with the door – my parents got to see their first-born child once again.

I suppose we all stayed up and chatted until about three o'clock that morning, with the older ones drinking tea and us eating the cakes and biscuits. Despite being our big sister, it felt at first as though we were strangers to Sister Chrys. Vincent was born three years after Fay left, so they had never met. Loretta was just three months old, I was three and Judy must have been about six when Fay left for Perth. We younger ones had long wondered about this sister who we'd only seen or remembered from photos, in the white habit of the hospital nurse and nun. The questions continued thick and fast. What was it like to be a nun? What about being a nurse? What's Perth like? Although she was exhausted after her long flight, Fay answered all of our questions and told us as much as she could about her life as a nun and her studies as a nurse. In the end it wasn't very long before we felt that she belonged and had always been there.

In the morning, after we woke, there was huge excitement, as there stood Fay in her full habit – black tunic, white veil, cap, wimple, the whole lot – which she had to wear during the day because she couldn't be seen without it, not even by her family walking around in their pyjamas. So over the next four weeks, we only saw her as a nun, even before breakfast when she sat in Mum's lovely rose garden saying the Divine Office. Mum was one of eight children, so we also had lots of uncles and aunts and other people coming to visit during Fay's stay, and while it went quickly, she was there for our baby sister Loretta's 13th birthday. Then three days later it was my 16th and another excuse for Mum's sponge cakes.

Over many other conversations during that visit, Fay told us – and reminded Mum – about the reasons why she had chosen to become a nun. She was just eight years old, asleep in her bed, when she had felt the presence of someone in the room. She told us she saw the vision of a man who kneeled beside her bed, made the sign of the cross over Fay, then blessed himself before standing and leaving the room. Fay said she'd told Mum about the vision the next morning but nothing more was said, as Mum thought it was probably a dream. Many years later, soon after she had joined the St John of God Convent in Subiaco, Fay was praying in the chapel when she looked up to see the face of the man who had come to see her and bless her as a child. It was the same face as that on the statue of St John of God. Fay's recollection of her vision stayed with me for many years as a reminder that, sometimes, you just know what you are meant to do.

4

MISTER SISTER

From a young age, I had always wanted to be a nurse, just like Fay and Coral or 'Codge' as we called her. I was always drawn to the idea of helping other people and being there for them when they needed it. As a 17-year-old, although I was the right age to enrol at Goulburn Base Hospital, they didn't accept male nurses. At the time, my only local trainee nursing option was Kenmore Psychiatric Hospital. Built in 1895, Kenmore is an historic asylum, the first purpose-built institution dedicated to mental health care in rural NSW, and is the largest example of the work of Australia's first Government Architect, W.L. Vernon. Dad took me to have a look at the huge, impressive complex on the outskirts of Goulburn, and while the staff kindly showed me around some of the wards, I decided this wasn't quite my idea of nursing. Instead, I went to work at Allens department store in Auburn Street, Goulburn, boarding with my auntie and uncle, who lived in my late maternal grandmother's house in the Goulburn suburb of Eastgrove. I got my driver's licence at 17 and, after working in the shoe department for a few years, I was able to save enough money to buy a new car, a shiny white Cortina, which set me back about $2000. Each weekend, my sister Judy and I would head to Cullerin to visit Mum and Dad, plus Loretta, then 15, and Vincent, 12. I slept in my old room and Judy shared a room with Ret.

One day, three years after the Kenmore visit, we went to Mass at St Brigid's as we always did on a Sunday morning. Back home, and after finishing our regular Sunday roast, Mum sat down to read the papers. 'Come and have a look at this, Keith,' she said, showing me an advertisement from Royal Prince Alfred Hospital in Camperdown, Sydney. The ad featured the crest of Prince Alfred and asked for applications for trainee nurses who wanted to become enrolled nurses. Alfred was Queen Victoria's second son who, during a visit to Australia in 1868, was shot in the back while on a picnic at Clontarf. The assassination attempt outraged members of the colony who opened a public subscription fund to build a hospital as a memorial to the prince's safe recovery. Alfred later authorised his coat of arms to be used as the hospital's crest and that symbol would become part of my life for almost half a century. The ad asked for applications from both males and females, with the training based at the hospital in Sydney. There was no nursing training at university in those days; it was all completed through a hospital. So my mother cut the coupon out of the paper and we filled in all the blanks – name, address, age, and so on – before she put it in an envelope, popped a stamp on it, franked the letter in our Cullerin post office and put it in the mailbag to be loaded onto the train to the Sydney GPO the next day.

About a fortnight later, back at Cullerin, Mum handed me an envelope featuring that now-familiar crest. It was a letter inviting me to attend Royal Prince Alfred Hospital for an interview. Several years earlier, my sister Loretta had also left home at 17 to start her nursing career at Lewisham Hospital in Sydney. While Ret loved the job, she had been very homesick and Vincent, Mum and I used to drive up the highway to her nurses' quarters on the occasional Sunday to visit her. Now here I was, a country boy in my new Cortina with my own passion to serve others, about to head off to the big smoke myself, hoping to secure a nursing job and not be too homesick.

In those days, Matron's Office at RPA was off to the side of the grand main entrance, but you entered via a side door which led into a small, simple waiting room featuring a few chairs and Matron's secretary seated behind a desk. It was all bathed in coloured light from one of the hospital's beautiful stained-glass windows. I was led into the main office and was greeted by Margaret Nelson, dressed in all her matronly glory – a crisply starched white uniform, long triangular veil, white stockings and sensible white shoes. Sister Olive, the Head of RPA's School of Nursing at the time, was also in the room, but dressed in a starched uniform of royal blue with a white veil, and beside her was another of the senior nursing staff, also in royal blue. I had always wanted to be a nurse, so this was my best opportunity to impress, and while I felt nervous, I answered all the questions throughout the interview and was fairly confident that I had done well. A couple of weeks later, a large envelope arrived at our post office.

You've been accepted into the Trainee Enrolled Nurses course and your starting date is April 9, 1970, wrote Matron Nelson.

The envelope also contained various instructions and another letter from Sister Olive outlining details of my accommodation, as all nurses had to live in back then. The main letter also stated that my first pay packet would be $36.10 – a fortnight! The salary was so poor that you really couldn't afford to live in Sydney in a flat or an apartment anyway, even with a bunch of friends, so on-site nurses' accommodation was the perfect solution.

On the way to begin my training, I stopped into Moss Vale to see Codge. It was her 32nd birthday and she was, by then, the mother of two children. While she is 12 years older than me, Codge had also been a big influence on my decision to become a nurse, so I needed her encouragement. When she first started a general training program at Berrima District Hospital, Codge would come home on her days off with tales about the hospital and her role in nursing, and I was intrigued by the stories about patients and how she cared for them. It was good to receive encouragement from Codge about the journey I was about to undertake.

Once I arrived at RPA, the letter from Sister Olive instructed me to report to the head sister at the nurses' home. The few males – one or two nurses and a nursing assistant – who needed a roof over their head were assigned to live on the first floor of the 1910 building. Who knows what would have happened if they'd let the men live in the same vicinity as the women! While a handful of men were at one end on the first floor, the other end housed quite a few female physios. The top floor of the building was reserved for male doctors.

My small room had quite a nice view over a tennis court and contained a desk, chair and wardrobe. The single bed had a plain wooden bedhead with a shelf, on which I put my portable alarm clock and my black, leather-bound transistor radio. The beds were so small that if you rolled over, you'd likely fall out. But I was used to a small bed, coming from such a large family and sleeping in a sliver of a bedroom for so long back at Cullerin. Next to the bed was a set of narrow French doors with a solid wood panel for the bottom half and a set of small windows at the top. The doors opened onto a shared verandah which later became the ideal spot to hang out as the rooms were too tiny to spend much time in. After a shift, we'd hit the verandah, catch up, chat and enjoy the fresh air. The only music would come from my transistor, as there were no power points in any of the rooms. If you wanted to plug in anything electrical, you had to trail a long extension cord down the hallway, then fight over one of the few sockets.

My written instructions had also indicated where I was to collect my uniform and a map showed me the way to the nurses' dining room, which had a broad verandah overlooking a beautiful square featuring a lovely stone fountain, which is still there today. I headed off to what was known as the sewing room to have my uniform fitted and discovered an ugly fibro building more than likely riddled with asbestos. The laundry room on the other side of the building had to do everything else in those days – wash all the nurses' uniforms, the doctors' gowns, patient gowns and all the bedding – so the building was huge. Our male nurses' uniform consisted of stiff white trousers and a sky-blue top with short sleeves. The collar was starched so it sat upright about an inch high around your neck. The male nurses' top was secured not by normal stitched-on buttons but by removable shiny plastic buttons secured on the inside by spring clips. You were told to remove the buttons and clips before putting your dirty uniform in the laundry, otherwise they'd go missing. The shirt had several pockets for all the bits and pieces required during a shift and while it was comfortable, the heavy drill cotton trousers were not.

In addition to this I always had to wear my new name badge, pinned to the left breast of my top. On it were etched the words 'TN Mr Dorsett Cox' which stood for Trainee Nurse, and my mother's maiden name – Dorsett. As there was more than one Cox at the hospital, the addition of your mother's maiden name helped distinguish you from the others. Mum had already sent away for little fabric strips with my name printed on them and she later stitched them to all five shirts and the waistbands of three pairs of trousers. Dirty uniforms would be deposited into a chute on each of the floors of our nurses' quarters, and the following day you'd head to the Laundry Room, tell them your name and they would locate your fresh uniform in one of the towering shelves marked A–Z. You would be handed a pile of clean, folded clothes and off you'd go, trailing a waft of freshly starched linen behind you. While our pay was a pittance, our board and meals were covered and we had the work laundry to take care of our washing, so it wasn't too bad.

The Queen Mary Building, now part of Sydney University student accommodation, housed the female nurses, who had single bedrooms featuring white or cream cabinetry made of tin rather than timber. They also shared a bathroom, a common room and a reading room on the ground floor. It was an impressive building, although not necessarily attractive, and consisted of ten floors. It also had a Grand Ballroom where we later enjoyed special dinners and Matron's annual Christmas lunch – which usually included a sneaky sherry or two, even if you were on shift.

I completed my 12-month trainee enrolled nurse's course, getting through without too much trouble, and our graduation was held in the ballroom. After my induction, I found that I was very passionate about nursing, and when you like something as much as this, you usually do well at it, so I wanted to learn more and was ready for whatever opportunity next presented itself.

Three of the people I met that year, John Bradley, a wardsman, his sister Margaret and their older brother Pat, a doctor, were New Zealanders. While I had settled in, John, whose room wasn't far from mine, was getting itchy feet. One day he said, 'Look, I'm jack of living in the nurses' home! Are you interested in getting a flat?'

Annoyed with sharing bathrooms and dining rooms and trailing extension cords up and down the corridor to get power to run my little record player, I offered him a resounding 'Yes'. So we looked around and eventually found a little place in Nelson Street, Annandale, an adjoining suburb. The flat had two bedrooms, a bathroom, a lounge–dining room with a balcony off it and a little kitchenette, as well as a shared laundry in the basement. It was in a good location as I could easily drive to RPA if needed and it was also within easy walking distance. While Pat had secured John a job, as he had for many other Kiwi compatriots, as a wardsman John earned even less than I did. As we were both on such poor wages, we asked Margaret and her friend Loretta Watson, who had the same first name as my sister, if they'd like to help share the rent. So, in 1971, we moved out of the old nurses' quarters and into our small flat.

By the time I became an enrolled nurse, a rare male at the time, I was on a bit more money. It was the early 1970s and I was living the inner-city life in Sydney with a bunch of nurses in their 20s. It wasn't hard for me to juggle work and partying like everyone else, even though I didn't drink much then, nor do I now. I'd often get home from a shift, even on a weekday, and there'd be a dozen people in our little two-bedder, drinking wine, having a laugh, listening to music or having a smoke on the balcony. We had some French guys living upstairs and one of them was very keen on Margaret, so he'd often come down to visit, always carrying a bottle of wine. Other friends were always popping in and out, and we'd often party on the weekend, especially if we all had Saturday off. My sister Loretta, who was still nursing at Lewisham Hospital, often came along, too, and it was at one of these parties that she met her future husband, Alan. Margaret had her 21st at the flat, as did I, but within six months of moving in we were evicted, given a week's notice because we were too noisy and all the neighbours had complained. Margaret and Loretta decided to head off to the eastern suburbs to live, while John, Pat and I found a nice garden flat in nearby Dulwich Hill. Everything I owned could fit into my car, so I packed it all into the boot and back seat of the Cortina and set off down New Canterbury Road.

The entry to our new digs was down a long driveway. It was a larger and more modern apartment than the Annandale flat and had a big lounge and dining area with glass doors opening out onto a garden. It also had an internal laundry, which was a novelty for me. While I stayed on at RPA as an enrolled nurse, John decided there was no future in being a wardsman, so he eventually returned to Christchurch where he enrolled in a geology degree. Pat and I recruited another flatmate, Val Turner, a doctor at RPA, and the three of us shared that Dulwich Hill flat for a while before Pat decided he'd buy a house in Ferry Road, Glebe. Pat and I moved to Glebe in 1973 with another of Pat's sisters, Christine. I didn't have a care in the world and although we were on minimum wage, they were happy days. I am still in contact with all of them, including Loretta Watson, then an assistant nurse who later made a decent living as a cook on the American TV show *Survivor*. John, meanwhile, is a professor and university lecturer in Hawaii, where he also works for NASA.

Even though I was happy with my new friends and my job, I was also experiencing a different kind of calling around this time. When I was young, I always wanted to be a nurse, but as my faith grew I thought God might have wanted me to do something else. My dad had converted to Catholicism, and my mother and her side of the family were quite religious. All of us kids were baptised, confirmed and went to Mass once a week, and faith was an important part of my life and my upbringing. But like anything, you have to work at it, and I continued to do so. I was influenced by another friend, Bob Slattery, who was then a nurse who also had a great devotion to Mary, mother of Jesus. Bob did gerontology first – the study of the social, cultural, psychological, cognitive and biological aspects of ageing – before becoming a registered nurse at the time when I was an enrolled nurse. We worked together on a ward and he and I became good mates because he had strong faith like I did, but his faith grew a lot more. He was older than me and knew the direction he wanted to go, and that was to St Paul's Seminary, in Kensington, which was for late vocations. 'Why don't you become a priest?' Bob said to me.

I was in my early 20s at the time and still an enrolled nurse, although not a registered nurse. While I wouldn't say I was slow to decide, I prayed a lot and went to Mass almost daily at St Joseph's in Missenden Road, near the hospital – hoping God would show me the way as I was a bit confused about my path. Then I said to Bob that I had a great devotion to St Francis of Assisi and I thought I'd like to be a Franciscan brother. So I started making enquiries and was told I needed to live in and experience the brotherhood as a novitiate at their training college in Campbelltown. After making more enquiries, I set off one day to see what it was like, but as soon as I got out there I thought, *This is not for me.* There were many interviews, vocational testing and so on, but I kept on hearing my dad's advice to Coral. At one point Codge had wanted to join a convent to follow in Fay's footsteps, but Dad had said: 'You can be a good Catholic and do good things without becoming a nun. I want you to think about this a bit longer, and then if you want to do it in a couple of years, you've got my blessing.'

The Franciscan order at Campbelltown was like being back on a farm, and there was a lot more praying than I expected, and brothers and priests wanting to chat about my faith. If I was to be a Franciscan brother, I didn't want to be working in the fields, I wanted to have more of that human touch. After the tests, they judged that I'd be reluctant to change that view and they didn't know if joining the Franciscans was the right thing for me to do. It was the right decision in the end. Dad's sage advice to Coral would also influence my final decision about my own career. After the Campbelltown experience, I visited Bob at the seminary and we had long discussions about faith and a calling. While he wasn't pushing me, he'd say: 'Why don't you go down the priesthood way?' But I don't think that was for me, either. I love patients and I love people, so it was nursing or nothing.

You can either grow in faith or you can just let it slide. I think I've been fortunate that even though I didn't take that path, I've also been able to grow in faith. Later, when I lived in the UK, I used to seek out the local Catholic church and go to Mass. Travelling through Europe for seven and a half months, I didn't always get to Mass, but the girls I travelled with were always on the lookout for me. 'Keith, there's a Catholic church here,' they'd say as we passed through a town or stopped for a break in a village somewhere, and I always checked the Mass times. They knew I was a churchgoer and neither they nor anyone else ever held it against me. Like-minded people often attract one another, I've found, and while the two girls I travelled with in the orange Kombi weren't Catholic, they were good people, and you don't have to be a Catholic to be a good person. Even though I didn't become a brother or priest in the end, I truly believe there are many different ways to live a life of service and I have continued to be involved in church and community throughout my life.

5

A FAMILY TRAGEDY

By 1974, my sister Loretta had married Alan, who she'd met at a party in our Annandale flat. I had been a groomsman at their wedding and we were all very close. They were living together in a small unit on Johnston Street, Annandale, with their baby daughter Kirsty, but they wanted a bit more room, so we all moved into a rental house in Young Street in the same suburb. I was being urged by RPA colleagues to undertake the three-year general nursing course, the next step up in my career, so I needed a bit more space myself. It wasn't long after we moved in that Ret, Alan and baby Kirsty headed off to Canberra to visit our sister Judy and her family. Judy had three children who had outgrown their baby walkers and bassinets and baby clothes which were destined for Kirsty. Ret worked the night shift Friday, Saturday and Sundays at Lewisham, and would finish early on Monday morning. As they left home at about 8 am that Monday, I remember waving them goodbye as I headed off to RPA.

After finishing my shift, I arrived back at our house and received a call from Alan's sister asking me to come over to their mother's place in St Peters. I knew something terrible had happened. I drove over and they were all in tears. They told me Loretta was in Royal Canberra Hospital but Alan and Kirsty were dead, killed in a car accident. Alan had been driving and Loretta was asleep in the front passenger seat, while Kirsty was in her bassinet in the back. Just before they were about to enter the ACT, Alan failed to take a bend in the road and had wrapped their Holden Commodore around a tree. Loretta woke in a daze to see Alan pinned behind the steering wheel, gasping for air. She then found Kirsty's tiny body at her feet and lifted her up to see a small scratch across the bridge of her baby's nose. But Kirsty was limp. Loretta looked at Alan again and watched him take his last few breaths. Loretta was covered in blood, had broken ribs, a broken arm and facial injuries, but managed to escape from the car, carrying Kirsty's body with her. Despite her injuries, the doctor at the hospital thought Loretta was stable enough to be collected by Judy and her husband, John.

'We'll stitch her up as best we can but we think she is better off going home with you tonight,' they told Judy before loading Loretta up with pain relief and sedatives.

Meanwhile, Alan and Kirsty were taken from the scene of the accident to the mortuary in Queanbeyan, where John was sent to identify their bodies. I flew down to Canberra the next day and John picked me up and took me straight to their home where I saw Loretta. It was the first real tragedy in my family and the first time I'd felt a real sense of helplessness. I felt I couldn't say or do anything to help Ret; all I could do was put my arms around her. When our dad arrived — and I still remember it so clearly – he gave Loretta the most beautiful hug, keeping control all the while.

'We all have a cross to bear in life but most people's crosses don't come this early. I'm so sorry,' he told her. But you could hear the emotion straining his voice. What I had learned after three years on the job was that to be a good nurse, you need to maintain a certain level of care. But you also need to have other qualities within yourself to do the job – like love and understanding – which are things that they don't teach you on the wards. So I took it upon myself to organise for the bodies of Alan and Kirsty to be sent to Sydney for the viewing and the funeral.

'I don't want any old wooden box for them,' Ret said to me. 'I want a nice coffin and they should be together.'

It might be considered unusual today but both my family and Alan's family wanted to see father and daughter one last time. The accident was so sudden and many of our relatives had not even met Kirsty, who was only five and a half months old when she died. So we dressed Alan in his wedding suit and Kirsty in her baptismal gown and both were laid out in the same coffin. The accident happened on a Monday and the funeral was held that Friday at their local church, St Brendan's in Annandale. Most of it was a blur, but what I do remember about the Mass was Ret asking me if she could take Communion, as if there was some reason why she couldn't or shouldn't. 'Yes, of course,' I said. Once we got to Rookwood Cemetery, Alan and Kirsty were laid to rest together, then we all went back to our now quiet Young Street house for the wake.

On the following Sunday, Loretta was admitted to Lewisham Hospital for further treatment for her injuries. The hospital had been established by the Sisters of the Little Company of Mary in the 1880s and they had developed it into a high-quality nursing facility. It had also been Loretta's training hospital, so there were many familiar faces there for her, including the remaining nuns. Within a few short hours of her return, the nuns had organised a 24-hour roster of all Ret's friends, plus volunteer nuns, to sit with her. They weren't there to help with her nursing or to do anything physical, just to be there with my sister in case she needed someone to talk to.

While Ret eventually returned to her regular shifts at Lewisham Hospital, for weeks and months afterwards, I'd hear her crying in our house in Annandale, but I felt helpless and couldn't ease her pain. The heartache is still there and always will be. I decided to put my career on hold as both families rallied to support Loretta through the ensuing months. My brother Vincent, by then a psychiatric nurse at Broughton Hall at Rozelle Hospital, had moved into our house in Annandale. So there we were, three siblings, all nurses, back in one house. But Loretta soon thought she needed more time to herself, so moved out with another nursing friend. After that brief pause, I started my general nursing course in January 1975.

6

DOING THE ROUNDS

Oncology was a new specialty and by 1977, although we didn't have a designated cancer ward, we did have 30 beds spread throughout RPA which were specifically for cancer patients. Twenty of those were in Blackburn Pavilion 4 (BP4) and BP5, and another ten were in other wards throughout the hospital. The Blackburn Pavilion was a standalone building connected by a walkway to the main hospital building. It had two wards, with the ground floor occupied by the central sterilising department, a floor of theatres, BP4 on the next floor and BP5, which was the haematology ward. In that year, when I was a third-year nurse, I met Professor Martin Tattersall, who had just been appointed the inaugural Chair of the new Cancer Medicine faculty at Sydney University, the first in the Southern Hemisphere. Martin was not only a Professor of Cancer Medicine and Head of Oncology at RPA, he was also head of the new Ludwig Institute, a research unit attached to Sydney University, which looked at new cancer treatment, new drugs and drug trials. Just 36 years of age when we met, the Yorkshireman had already been a research fellow at Marsden Hospital in the UK, a visiting fellow at Harvard Medical School and the Dana-Farber Cancer Institute in the US, and a consultant physician at Charing Cross Hospital, London. He had also completed a PhD in Boston on the use of the drug methotrexate to treat cancer, which was usually prescribed for rheumatoid arthritis. Martin had used it in the treatment of US Senator Edward M. Kennedy's 12-year-old son, Edward M. Jr, who'd already had his right leg amputated above the knee to halt bone cancer. Martin was convinced methotrexate cured the boy of the disease.

After I finished my general nursing training in January 1978, I was awarded the Hospital Medal for Outstanding Achievement, the only male nurse ever to be given that honour. It's a record that still stands as the Hospital Medal no longer exists and nursing training now takes place at university. I was also sent a letter in beautiful copperplate writing on personal letterhead by veteran surgeon and former president of the Royal Australasian College of Surgeons, Professor Sir John Loewenthal, after I received the Hospital Medal on graduation.

Dear Mr Dorsett-Cox,

I have just heard that you have been awarded the proficiency medal and wanted to offer you our warm congratulations. I have appreciated your thoughtful and sensitive care of my patients — especially Mrs Munch & am delighted that the high standard of your work is being recognised.

Yours very kindly

JS Loewenthal

After becoming an RN, I went to work as a ward sister on Blackburn Pavilion 4, which was renowned for its heavy workload. The weekly rounds were always conducted on a Tuesday and ours were always at 9 am. The medical team included a professor of surgery, various other specialist surgeons, registrars and residents, plus an intern and physiotherapist and, on occasion, a social worker and a registered nurse, which was now me. So I would accompany the team on the rounds, sometimes a baker's dozen of us, a daily file up and down the ward to see the patients. As ward sister, I carried a ledger of all patients which revealed their name, age and what was wrong with them, along with the name of their surgeon. On the far right of the ledger was another column where I could jot down instructions and the doctor's orders for the patients: 'Mrs Smith can have her drain removed', or 'Mr Jones can have his bandage changed', or 'Mrs Wright could get up and move around and walk today' or 'start ambulating' as the doctors would like to say.

After our troupe did the rounds of the wards – which took about 40 minutes to an hour, depending on how many patients there were and how many questions they would ask – there was time for a tea break. There was a sunlit room on the floor known as 'the solarium', a very Victorian name for a room full of windows, not for sunbaking as it may imply. Tables and comfortable chairs overlooked the tennis court and the old non-denominational chapel outside. It was quite a pleasant room and both patients and nursing staff used to enjoy it – but not at the same time – having a quiet coffee or being able to take a short breather from the ward. In those days, the nurses' dining room was in the Queen Mary Building, which was too far away to be able to enjoy any significant break before you were required back on the ward. But if you were a ward sister, as I was, you could head off the ward to the dining room in the 1936 Sisters' Home for lunch. It was free in those days, and if you got there early enough, there was quite drinkable tea made with several spadefuls of Kinkara or Billy Tea stewing away in a large urn. But if you got there late, which I did more often than not, the tea turned into this horrible dark brown liquid the colour of treacle, and offered nothing more than a tarry, burnt taste on the tongue. It turned me off tea for good, so I took to having a spoonful of International Roast from the tin, accompanied by the occasional finger bun.

While I had already decided to head overseas on an extended working holiday, after several months on BP4, the charge sister decided to leave, and I was encouraged by several colleagues, including Martin Tattersall and the section's assistant director of nursing, Sister 'Rossie' Ross McPherson, to apply for the position, even though I was just 28, not long out of general training and considered quite young to take over a hospital ward. I wouldn't say I was inexperienced – I had been nursing for eight years by then, and I did show some leadership potential that professors Loewenthal and Tattersall, and vascular surgeon Michael Stephen, some other doctors and even one senior nurse must have recognised. Even though all who supported me understood that I was going overseas the following year, I was still encouraged to apply for the position. But, at the time, I had other ideas about my career path, and it wasn't in cancer. Back then, cancer nursing was known for its patients being constantly sick from primitive treatment and also having a very poor recovery rate. I was focused on a career in accident and emergency or intensive care because I liked 'drama' nursing, as it was called. But my lack of appreciation for cancer nursing would later change.

In mid-1978, I was appointed charge sister of BP4, taking it on with the understanding that I would only be there for ten months as I wanted to embark on that rite of passage for many young Australians – a working holiday to England and Europe, which I had planned with some other nurses at RPA, Barb and Belinda. Professor Loewenthal had even provided me with a glowing personal reference to use for job applications in London, and Professor Tattersall and another oncologist, Dr Bob Woods, both thought I'd make a good cancer nurse and had also provided me with references. You never look a gift horse in the mouth, so if someone wants to give you a glowing reference then you graciously accept it.

It was around that time that I met a young man called Chris O'Brien, who was a surgical registrar on BP4. He stood out even then, not only because of his charisma but because he was a very nice, personable young man. He was intelligent, a good communicator, and I found him to be unlike the other doctors I knew at the time who were mostly of the old school. I am a people person, I suppose, and Chris was a good people person too. He was kind to the patients and nice to the staff so was an all-round great guy. He was also a man of faith, Roman Catholic like me, a churchgoer, and our strong beliefs were the same. We also had a similar understanding of our place in the world, so it was no surprise that our approach to medicine was quite similar, too. We both felt we had been born to serve. We got to know each other fairly well over that brief period and just before I was ready to leave for the UK, I had a farewell party. While a few others gave speeches, including professors and nurses, Chris ended up giving the speech on behalf of the whole medical team.

While I was in the UK from 1979–81 – my one and only absence from RPA in my entire professional career – Chris finished his surgical registrar training and continued work on his specialty of head and neck surgery. The allure of London was also strong for him and he too headed to the UK for further studies, a long-accepted tradition for career-focused young Australian doctors.

When I think back to my early years of nursing in the 1970s and 80s, what I remember is that even though there was plenty of hard work and learning, we also managed to have a lot of fun. Some of the stories from that time likely wouldn't (and shouldn't) happen in today's nursing environment, but they helped keep our spirits up in what could be a difficult job.

LIKE A BUDGIE IN A CAGE

Vascular surgeon Michael Stephen was one of the well-known characters on the medical team during my time at RPA as a ward sister. He had a very particular opening routine and would come up to the bedside of each patient, stand there and put his hand out to greet them.

'Congratulations! You've done so well after this operation,' he'd say. 'It was very hard, it was a very difficult surgery but look how well you've done. Look at you today!'

After a while, I'd know exactly what Dr Stephen would say, reeling off the same speech, time and again – unless the patient hadn't recovered so well, of course. As it all got rather predictable, I decided to play a practical joke on him and one particular Tuesday on our rounds, I had a few words with the first couple of patients before Dr Stephen started off. He approached the first patient, as usual, poked his hand out and was about to launch into his speech when the patient piped up: 'Congratulations, Dr Stephen, I've done so well after this operation. It was very hard, it was a very difficult surgery but look how well I've done. Look at me today!' And we all broke up laughing. He took it well. Then he approached the next patient and the same speech came back to him, like a budgie in a cage. My coaching certainly broke the monotony of the ward rounds that day.

WHERE THERE'S SMOKE...

While just about everyone smoked back then, both pipes and cigarettes, it wasn't supposed to be done inside the wards, on a doctor's rounds, or next to patients. But Dr Stephen, who had dubbed me 'Dors', an abbreviation of my hospital name, 'Dorsett', used to absent-mindedly bring his pipe with him, puffing away as he strolled into the ward. So I'd tell him off. 'Michael! Put that away!' I'd say. So he'd place his thumb over the top of the pipe to snuff out the embers of the tobacco and then pop it into his pants pocket. On one particular occasion, he walked in, pipe in mouth, saw me, heard my usual 'Michael! Put that away!' and did exactly what I told him. But a few minutes later, in the middle of our rounds, there was an odd odour. 'Can you smell that?' someone said. It was Michael's pipe and the smell was of burning tobacco and a trouser pocket which had caught on fire! I dare say he never did that again.

THREE SHEETS TO THE WIND

Hospital work and nursing, in particular, used to be quite regimented, reflecting its military origins. You wore a clean uniform and changed your top every day and your pants every second day. You couldn't wear a cardigan or jumper, and any jewellery, such as watches or bracelets, was banned because of the risk of contamination. You couldn't even sit on a bed and talk to a patient, as you can now. Nurses knew their place and it was a fair way down the ladder behind doctors and surgeons. But things were also a lot more relaxed in many ways. We were always able to have a bit of fun, both during our shift and after work. One of the more adrenaline-charged activities involved riding a stainless-steel trolley on casters down a hospital ward. Known as a dressing trolley, it was loaded with new bedding and each night we'd restock the top and bottom decks with clean linen which was destined for the patients' beds the following morning. So, for a bit of a thrill, we'd pack the upper deck with linen and enough room for a nurse to lie flat out on top, then we'd put the remaining linen on the bottom shelf. Then another nurse would give the dressing trolley a good heave-ho down the ward and patients and nurses would watch this stainless-steel trolley, piloted by a flying nurse, go careering down the length of the room – and this was one very long ward.

HIGH-RISE COMMODE

During my many ward rounds – I must have walked a million miles – there were some particularly memorable incidents that you may find hard to believe. On one occasion in 1978 when I was charge sister of BP4, the attending doctor, Michael Stephen, had made a note on the ledger giving one female patient commode privileges. She was on bed rest but the privilege meant she could now use a portable toilet rather than a bedpan. In the normal course of events, that meant putting a commode next to the bed, so a patient could relieve themselves without having to walk down the corridor to the bathroom. One nurse, just out of preliminary training school, was given the job of organising the commode and toileting the patient. On our next ward visit, Dr Stephen and I were approaching the bay when the patient's head popped up a few inches above the six-foot-high curtain. 'Hi,' says the patient, obviously pleased with herself but oblivious to the danger. We pulled back the curtain to reveal she was balancing precariously on a commode strapped to the end of her bed. The trainee nurse had somehow combined bed rest and commode privileges and lifted the portable toilet – which comprised a heavy steel chair and stainless-steel pan – onto the end of the bed, securing it with crepe bandages.

'*Dors!* What's going on here?' Dr Stephen demanded to know. I was quite embarrassed but had no answers. We were both astonished that not only had the nurse put the commode on the bed, but the patient had participated in the high-wire act as well.

FANGS FOR THE MEMORIES

Just a few decades ago, most of our elderly patients had false teeth. Because of fewer visits to the dentist and no fluoride in the water, the removal of all your teeth, worn, rotten or not, was not uncommon. In the late 1970s, a young nurse with her own lovely original smile was given the task of approaching each of the elderly patients and asking them to hand over their dentures so they could be scrubbed and cleaned. Rather than do it one at a time, the nurse collected all of the dentures from the whole ward, placed them in one dish and proceeded to clean the lot, scrubbing away with a little brush. She was pleased with her work and the efficiency of this process. However, after she was done she realised she hadn't had the foresight to label each set of dentures, and having no idea which set belonged to whom, she was then forced to go to each hospital bed, frantically holding up several sets of unidentified dentures in front of the elderly patient's face, asking the now bewildered and still toothless recipient: 'Do these belong to you?'

WARM-BLOODED

Most blood transfusions are given over two to three hours, but if a patient with an underlying medical condition requires a faster transfusion, the blood usually needs to be warmed during administration. One fourth-year nurse, who in those days had four stars on her cap as a mark of her seniority, told a trainee nurse that the patient needed a faster transfusion. Blood transfusions always need to be checked by two nurses, both via label checks as well as confirming the name, date of birth and blood type with the patient. With this particular warming method, you set a bag of blood on the IV pole, then you attach what is called a 'blood giving set' to the end of another standard giving set which is then connected to an electronically warmed water bath, into which the blood is redirected via a coil. This was in the late 1970s, in the Page Chest Pavilion where Lifehouse now stands, and the trainee nurse was instructed to make sure she warmed the blood. Having never done it before, the trainee nurse disappeared down the ward to complete the task. Before this particular transfusion, the trainee nurse decided to do things a bit differently. She found a saucepan in the kitchen, tore open the plastic bag of blood, poured the contents into the saucepan and put it on the hotplate where she proceeded to warm it up. Needless to say, the hot blood in the saucepan had to be thrown out. It just shows that you should never assume someone knows what to do, so from then on I made sure each nurse understood every instruction!

LET THEM EAT CAKE

During my time in BP4, one of the oncologists, Derek Raghavan, came along to the Tuesday ward round with one of his registrars.

'I've made cake,' the registrar said proudly. She put her cake down on the table in the meeting room before the ward round and we cut it and all had a piece. She went on and on about the numerous ingredients, how difficult it was to make and what effort it had taken. Derek popped it in his mouth, took a meaningful chew and rolled it around thoughtfully. 'That's a six!' he finally piped up, as if scoring a Torvill and Dean performance. At the time, the English ice skaters had a habit of achieving perfect scores, which were marked out of six.

The next Tuesday, a resident doctor arrived before our rounds carrying a homemade cake, trying to outdo the registrar. And that proved the start of our cake competition. Each Tuesday, someone would be rostered on to bring in a cake, and every week we'd see increasingly lavish cakes often decorated in icing with a theme related to a cancer treatment. While Martin Tattersall loved the cakes, he was always running late, had too many things to do and too much on his plate to make his own. When it came time for him to present his baked goods, we all presumed he would fail to deliver. But there he was on his rostered Tuesday, cake thrust on the table, a magnificent fruity

creation with the word *harringtonine* – a cancer drug – carefully spelled out in hundreds-and-thousands on his icing-free
jam-glazed fruitcake.

I don't know whether this is true or not, even to this day, but
the story goes that the night before the cake was due, he got
home and said to his wife, Sue: 'I'm on for the cake tomorrow!'

'You didn't tell me you were on for cake,' said Sue, who also
had a lot on her plate with her job as a respiratory physician
at North Shore Hospital, quite apart from being the mother
of three boys and the wife of Martin Tattersall. 'Do you have
any ingredients for a cake?' Martin asked somewhat desper-
ately, foraging around their kitchen. 'No, because you didn't
tell me you needed them,' she said, increasingly exasperated. So,
out he went, late at night, scrambling around trying to find a
shop that was open and would sell a half-crazed man eggs and
flour and icing sugar. He decided to head down to Haymarket,
right in the heart of the Sydney CBD, as he knew it was always
buzzing at night so he'd find something open there. As he was
walking around trying to find some ingredients – although still
undecided on what he was going to bake and how he was
going to decorate it – a fellow approached him. The man said:
'I saw you on TV! You were talking about a new chemotherapy
drug called harringtonine.' Suddenly inspired by this stranger,
Martin knew what he was going to do. 'That,' he said to himself,
'is the cake I'm going to present tomorrow.'

So he found a little mini-mart and bought all the ingredients
for a fruitcake, which he thought would suit everyone – dried
fruit and eggs and butter and flour, possibly all well past their
use-by date. Back at home, he got the cake in the oven and, of
course, it took hours to cook. So he ate his dinner late that night,

watching and waiting for his fruitcake to bake, and knowing he would then have to decorate it.

The next day, triumphant that he had fooled us all by managing to create a cake, Martin waxed lyrical with the long and involved story of his masterpiece, and the high degree of difficulty required to create this work of art, and as the story was strung out and the embellishment got even greater, he was expecting a high score. Well, we all judged the cake – and the accompanying story – but Martin didn't rate that well. I only ate a small piece, but a few hours later those who had indulged in the meeting room fruitcake kept disappearing off to the bathroom. Then a queue began forming outside the toilets. 'What's wrong?' I asked one of the unfortunates. 'It must be something I ate,' she responded.

Other cakes came thick and fast. In the 1990s, at E9 Special Unit, Derek Raghavan was preparing to leave us to take up a position as head of oncology at a hospital in the US. As a farewell gesture, he dressed in a white suit similar to that of a cruise ship steward and sported an old-fashioned bright orange lifejacket. The cake he presented was of a sinking ship and the picture I still have shows him looking crestfallen, as if he were disappointed that he was abandoning the good ship RPA. Another to 'jump ship' and present a cake was Professor Michael Friedlander. Michael's version was of a dinosaur (us at RPA) on one piece of land, and a toy car crossing a Toblerone bridge to the lurid 'greener pastures' of Sydney's North Shore, where cows and a horse were grazing.

7

NOT SO LUCKY THE
SECOND TIME AROUND

By 1979 all nine of us Cox kids had left home and were scattered around the country, from my brothers still in Goulburn to my sister Fay, Sister Chrys, now a nun, midwife and paediatric nurse who was living and working with Aboriginal communities on reserves all around Western Australia. I was already well entrenched at RPA and at BP4 with European travel plans formulating in my head.

It was early one morning in late January, about six months before I was due to leave for England, when I received a telephone call at home telling me I needed to get to Goulburn as soon as possible. Mum and Dad had been hurt during a robbery at our Cullerin home, I was told. I must have been in shock as I said I'd head down as soon as I could but needed to go to work first to sort a few things out. Being in charge of a ward, you can't just up and leave. So I went straight to the hospital and told my boss what had happened and why I needed to leave so urgently. I was doing the things I needed to do before handing over to my second-in-charge when surgeon Michael Stephen spotted me. The assault and robbery had already made the morning news, and most people in the hospital had heard.

'What are you doing here, Dors?' he asked. 'Wasn't it your parents who were assaulted?'

'Yes, I'm just tying up these few things then I'm out of here,' I told him.

My friend Belinda drove me down to Goulburn Base Hospital and that was where I found Mum and Dad together in a two-bedded room. I remember walking in and just bursting into tears, shocked to see the faces of my elderly parents bruised, battered and almost unrecognisable. My father was black and blue from the top of his head to his chest. His jaw was broken in three locations. My mother's false eye – she had been accidentally blinded in her right eye with a pencil by her sister when she was young – was pushed right back into the socket and she also had a large haematoma (medical speak for a bruise) on her right cheekbone, which they had to drain from the inside. Mum also had bruises and lacerations across her face. She was just getting over a cholecystectomy, too, having had her gall-bladder removed several weeks prior, so was lucky not to have split open her surgical wounds.

I slowly pieced together what had happened. As was his habit, Dad had been sitting at the end of the breakfast table doing the books and eating a late dinner my mother had prepared. It was 10 pm and Mum was in bed, while Dad had all the daily takings piled up on the table, alongside the ledger in which he recorded all the incomings and outgoings from the petrol station, post office, general store and poultry farm. Dad was meticulous with his bookwork and was so engrossed in the ledger and his dinner that he failed to see two men standing over him until he heard their voices. It didn't help that he was hard of hearing by this stage. One of the pair started grabbing all the money from the table while the other demanded to know where the rest of the cash was. Police suspected they had been watching the shop for a couple of days and knew Dad hadn't been to Goulburn to bank the money, so it had to be in the house somewhere. But not even my mother knew where Dad hid the cash. None of us knew. Dad had built the post office himself by hand, so the stash could have been anywhere.

The men started bashing my poor dad, demanding to know where the money was, but he refused to say. Then one of them headed to my parents' bedroom and grabbed my mum, holding a knife to her throat. The first thing she thought was, *If they start hitting me, my surgery wounds will open up*, and she tried to wriggle across the bed, but the intruder kept hold of her and started bashing her around the face. No doubt Dad knew Mum was putting up a struggle in the other room while he was also copping a hiding. When Mum did manage to get across the double bed, she was lying sideways still kicking away at this thug when she heard the other man say: 'Come on, I've got it,' and with that, they grabbed all the cigarettes out of the shop, plus the rest of the takings from Dad's hidden location, before stealing his car keys and driving off into the night.

After they left, Mum staggered to her feet and went to find my father, feeling her way down the hall as she was half-blinded by all the blood from her facial injuries. When she reached Dad, he was tied up and bleeding profusely. The thugs had upturned a chair, cut the cord from the iron and tied Dad with it, continuing to bash him while demanding to know where the rest of the cash was.

'I'll go and ring the police,' Mum said, but Dad stopped her, fearing the thugs might still be around. After she managed to set Dad free, they both went to the post office to make the call but the thieves had cut the main telephone line to the shop. My father said: 'I'll go for help,' and my mother said: 'No, I'll go for help,' with both of them standing there covered in blood and the whole house looking like a murder scene. So they switched on all the shop lights and were about to head outside to the red public telephone box when they caught a very lucky break. Dad always left a can of water up at the bowsers so truckies could fill up whenever they needed, day or night. That very evening, a semitrailer driver just happened to have stopped to get water when he saw all the shop lights come on and looked down to see my parents, standing there covered in blood.

'We've been assaulted and robbed and they've cut the phone line,' my mother told the truckie through a veil of bloody tears.

'What about the telephone box?' said the truckie, and went over to check the line. It worked, so he called an ambulance and then the police, who phoned Ronnie in Goulburn as well as my other brother Brian, and both sped out to Cullerin. By the time my brothers arrived, the paramedics were putting our parents into the back of an ambulance. Brian later said that when he entered our home, there was blood everywhere, from the breakfast room to the dining room, from the bathroom to the bedroom, in the kitchen and the hall, and trailing through to the shop. Our post office included a timber service counter with a glass screen, under which you slid money and letters and parcels. Under that counter and screen, Dad had built all these cupboards, about six inches square – little pigeonholes each featuring a local family name written across the top. The Joneses had one pigeonhole assigned to them for their mail, then the Smiths, and so on. We later found out that at the bottom of all these pigeonholes was a false floor under which Dad hid the takings after squaring the ledgers late at night, well after everyone else had gone to bed. It was only after they'd bashed him to within an inch of his life and also beaten my mother that he'd revealed where it was. When the police arrived they took fingerprints where they could find them.

After we had all left home, Mum and Dad had acquired a little poodle called Sammy and he was like their tenth child, spoiled and allowed to sleep on their bed. While Sammy wasn't touched during the robbery and assault, he was badly shaken, so after Brian and his wife Joyce cleaned up the house they took a frightened and quivering Sammy home to Goulburn with them. The following article on the assault of Bill and Pansy Cox appeared in the *Canberra Times* on 26 January 1979.

Alert for two men after elderly couple attacked

Police in Goulburn have issued an alert for two young men travelling in a stolen utility, after assaults on an elderly man and his wife at Cullerin, near Goulburn.

The police said the couple were viciously attacked in their home after closing their general store on Wednesday night.

Two men, thought to be in their early 20s, forced their way inside about 10 pm, threatened the couple with a knife, took a wallet of money and some loose cash from the house, and bashed both victims about the head.

The man, aged about 75, and his wife, about 67, are in
Goulburn Hospital with head injuries. Police said they have not
been able to interview the man, who may have a broken jaw.

By the time I got to Goulburn Base Hospital the next morning, the police had already caught the two crooks in Crookwell, about 40 minutes drive north-east of Cullerin, and had recovered Dad's car, a very distinctive canary-yellow Ford Falcon utility. What the perpetrators didn't appreciate was that our family was well known in the area, my father in particular. These guys had also taken off in an easy-to-spot bright yellow ute, driven it from Cullerin to Crookwell, then dumped it in a side street before heading to a café to have breakfast, no doubt to be paid for with their ill-gotten gains. After walking through the door of the café, they ordered tea and a big breakfast before asking for directions out of town.

'What's the quickest way to get to Dubbo?'

The café proprietor had already heard about the break-in and bashing of the Coxes at Cullerin on the radio news that morning and thought these guys fitted the bill.

'I've just got to go get more milk. Are you guys right for a minute?' he said to them.

'Yes, that's fine,' they replied as he headed out the front door of the café then spotted Dad's yellow ute up the road. So the café proprietor went into the greengrocer next door. 'Phone the cops,' he said. 'I've got the two guys who bashed the Coxes in my shop. I'm cooking them bacon and eggs for breakfast, so they'll be there for a while.' Then he grabbed some milk and headed back to the café.

'Sorry to keep you waiting,' he told the pair, 'I'll have breakfast for you in a jiffy.' But before they even got to sip their tea and enjoy their bacon and eggs, the police arrived to arrest them.

When I arrived at Goulburn Base Hospital with Belinda, the nursing staff were almost ready to take Dad to Canberra Hospital for surgery on his broken jaw. After he left in the ambulance, my brothers and their wives and Belinda and I sat with Mum, who was on painkillers and still very groggy from the assault. A few hours later, we headed back to Cullerin where we were met by my other friend Kim, who had driven down from Sydney despite having a wisdom tooth extracted that very morning. Belinda, Kim and I had to spend the night somewhere, and as my brothers had already cleaned up the house and shop, we decided to stay there. We nurses weren't afraid of the sight of blood, which had already been cleaned up in any case, and the culprits were already locked up, but that night we all slept fitfully and armed ourselves with weapons: me with a lump of wood and Belinda a pair of wooden clogs which were very much in fashion in operating theatres at the time. Spooked by the incident and the isolation, we all woke at the slightest noise, whispering across the corridor: 'What was that?', weapons raised.

The injuries inflicted by a callous pair of cowards who bashed and robbed an elderly, hard-working couple were severe. There followed various surgeries and hospital stays over a long period, a slow and painful process for my parents and one from which they never completely recovered. Dad was in Canberra Hospital for almost a month but even after three surgeries, and hindered by bad arthritis, his jaw never fully healed. As his health declined, Dad used to say to me: 'It's all these anaesthetics that are causing this.'

Mum was taken to Sydney Eye Hospital to have her eye socket rebuilt, with surgeons taking the mucosal lining from the inside of her cheek to rebuild it so she could put her glass eye back in. The Cullerin shop, meanwhile, had to be shut because Mum and Dad were in no fit state to run it and we kids couldn't either. It was a relentless 12-hour-a-day, seven-day-a-week operation. None of us was in a position where we could just pack up our lives and leave to run a country store, post office, petrol station and farm. Mum stayed with Brian and Joyce for a month or so while Dad was in the hospital, but as soon as he had recovered enough, Dad returned home and re-opened the shop. Although Cullerin had been our home and a place of business for 40-odd years, Mum never felt safe there again and hated returning to live at the back of the shop. She would have got up and left anytime, given the opportunity. Added to that, Mum and Dad were in their 60s and 70s by then and didn't need to work. They could have gone on the pension. But the shop was their life and Dad, in particular, didn't want to take money from the government – which is how he saw it – insisting on continuing to run the business.

'What else are we going to do?' he would say. But us kids would plead with him: 'Dad, you don't need to work, none of us wants the business, although we know it's hard for you to comprehend that. We've seen how you worked. You never had holidays or even a day off. We don't want that lifestyle.'

I left for Europe soon after, despite my concerns for my parents' welfare. During my absence overseas, one of the pair that had attacked and robbed my parents was jailed for five years with a non-parole period of three years while the other received a three-year sentence with a non-parole period of

18 months. As a man of faith, I had to learn to forgive those who had committed this crime against my loved ones. I was very angry at first, and I didn't forgive them straight away. But I did eventually forgive. As they say, 'Love thy neighbour', and I believe that living this way has helped me to find peace and share my love with not just one person, but many.

8

APPOINTMENT AT THE ROYAL MARSDEN

When I first arrived in England with Barb and Belinda, the three of us wrote out a lot of job applications and sent off many letters to several hospitals in the UK, because we wanted some work to come back to after our European tour. We were about to use up all our savings touring the UK for a month, then spend six weeks on the road in Europe in our bright, left-hand-drive Kombi – dubbed the Orange Baron, with a toy Snoopy riding on the dash – meeting old friends and making new ones. Our trip included the rites of passage for any Australian of that era: the Running of the Bulls in Pamplona, the Munich Oktoberfest, and joining a gypsy caravan of three other Kombis which held more than a dozen travellers in all. We searched for a beach in Greece to camp out on and lived on what little money we had, spending balmy summer evenings cooking fresh fish over open campfires. By the time I returned to London, I was broke and the clothes on my back were falling apart from being washed in the salty waters of the Mediterranean. But happily, the responses to our letters and job applications were waiting for us in a mailbox I had set up at Australia House. I was accepted at both a hospital in Bath to do my ICU training, and at another hospital for A&E training. I was also encouraged to come in for an interview at the Royal Marsden, by then a well-known cancer hospital next to the Royal Brompton Hospital in the salubrious Kensington and Chelsea district. The Marsden seemed very casual and low-key, and although I'd thought it would be a proper job interview, it seemed more like a quick chat.

'So, when did you want to interview me?' I said at the end of our little talk.

'Oh, you've just had your job interview. You can start whenever you like,' was the reply.

The cancer nurses' course started in just one month's time, but I didn't have any money left after Europe, so I needed to earn some before starting any course. I also needed to get my head around studying again, so I delayed starting the course and continued working as a casual agency nurse until the following May, six months later.

The Marsden was the first hospital in Europe to specialise in cancer treatment. It was small – the wards held a maximum of 24 beds – and the staff seemed to have the patients' best interests at heart, much more so than the other larger hospitals I had been to in London. When I first I started at the Marsden, I thought: *I like this, I like the feel, I like the delivery of care.* I liked the newness of oncology and the search for knowledge about the subject. And most of all I thought: *This is going to be my specialty!*

My cancer nursing certification would take nine months, and included three months consolidation to complete it, which was a commitment to working at the Marsden after my training. While it is based in London, the Marsden has another hospital in Sutton, in Surrey, which is where I completed the last three months of my course. Even if you weren't living in the nurses' quarters at the Marsden, they offered you free accommodation in Surrey, so I could not only live in Sutton during my shifts, but I could also continue to share the flat in London with my friends. If I went elsewhere, to another regional hospital, I would have had to leave all my friends and I wanted to stay in London, so the Royal Marsden was the ideal solution.

While there are many stories from my time at the Royal Marsden, one of my favourites is about a guy named Jimmy. I'd completed the oncology course at the Marsden and was finishing my consolidation on the Wilson Ward – half of which was head and neck cases and the other half was 'gynie' (gynaecological cases). Jimmy was in one of the head and neck rooms and he had larynx cancer. His background, as was the case with a lot of head and neck patients, was that of a heavy drinker and smoker, and despite his condition he would still partake of our regular drinks trolley – and then some – each evening. A portion of whisky would be poured down Jimmy's nasogastric tube via a Toomey syringe. To complete this process, we would take the nozzle off the syringe, put it over the tube and inject the whisky. Jimmy couldn't taste it as it was going down, of course, as it was nowhere near his tongue, but the alcohol would have the same effect it always did and Jimmy would get the fumes as they were belched back up.

Jimmy had already had some quite extensive surgery, including the removal of his voice box as well as his lymph glands as a result of his metastatic disease. Now, those particular glands are quite close to the carotid artery, and as Jimmy had also undergone radiotherapy, which had made his skin paper-thin, it wasn't a good combination. When I arrived early one morning for my 7 am shift, I was told that Jimmy had blown his carotid artery during the night and had been in danger of bleeding out. His artery had burst through his skin, spraying blood across the room. They were still cleaning up when I got there and the evidence was everywhere to be seen − blood on the walls, the curtains, even on the ceiling. I was told that when the carotid had burst, a quick-thinking and creative senior nurse had put her fist into Jimmy's neck in an attempt to stop the haemorrhage. While she kept her fist jammed in there to stem the flow of blood, she had instructed a junior nurse to grab a cuffed trache-ostomy tube. This tube is usually placed down the windpipe and a small balloon is inflated via a syringe, to keep the tube from falling out of the trachea. The senior nurse had managed to put one of these tubes into Jimmy's carotid artery, blown the cuff up and had been able to stem the bleeding. Jimmy was then rushed to the operating theatre where surgeons spent the night repairing the burst artery. I was a young nurse and while I had some experience, I would never have thought of grabbing a cuffed tracheostomy tube as an option. Being creative saved a life that night.

Jimmy was in intensive care after that, being fed via a naso-gastric tube. But after a couple of days he was returned to Wilson Ward where he recovered enough to be sent back to his home in Jersey.

'Have you ever been to Jersey?' I was asked. 'No,' I said. 'Well,' came the reply, 'Jimmy needs a nurse escort to take him back there.'

What a great idea, I thought, and agreed to the proposal, looking forward to a free mini holiday to a place I'd never been. They booked a flight for Jimmy and me for the following Saturday morning. Jimmy could walk by then but was very thin, had a nasogastric tube poking out of his nostril and bandages on his neck where the carotid artery had blown and, of course, his trachie tube. In short, he looked a mess. I also assumed that he had some brain damage from the episode when his carotid had blown as blood had stopped flowing to his brain for a brief period. We were travelling in a small plane, maybe a 50-seater, sitting side by side, and had priority boarding. We were buckled up, waiting for everyone else to board, when Jimmy started making some grunting noises and pointing his thumb downward in the direction of his tube, making 'glug, glug' sounds. It was only about 11 am but he wanted a drink.

'Can't you try and control your father?' the stewardess asked me. Well, that got my blood boiling. I flushed with embarrassment.

'He is *not* my father,' I said brusquely. It was the first time in my career that I wished I had worn my uniform in public. 'I am a nurse and I'm escorting him back home to Jersey.'

'Well, he's going to have to wait until we've taken off before he gets anything to drink.'

'Jimmy, you are going to need to hang five until we take off,' I repeated to my charge. Soon after the plane was in the air, Jimmy started making noises again and the stewardess offered him two of those little 50-millilitre bottles of whisky. 'That's enough,' I told the stewardess. Knowing Jimmy, I had packed a Toomey syringe and we 'administered' one mini bottle of whisky, then the second. But he wanted more and kept on making the 'glug, glug' sign with his thumb pointing down his tube.

Fortunately, it was a short flight, and when we landed soon after, there was someone from Jersey General Hospital waiting for us. My duty of care did not finish until I'd got Jimmy from hospital door to hospital door, so we took the supplied car to Jersey General where I felt no qualms in handing over both Jimmy and his paperwork. Bravo, we had made it. I spent Saturday night having a brief look around, going out to dinner at the local pub before heading back to my hotel. The following morning, I jumped on a plane back to London.

Throughout those three months of consolidation training, the medical staff were fabulous and they were all willing to teach me new things. The senior nurses were particularly fantastic. Robert Tiffany was the chief nursing officer then and he'd written several medical books for nurses, a rarity in the late 1970s and early 1980s. He was put on a pedestal by all of the nursing staff and was later knighted for this work. Richard Wells was another standout. He was a nursing officer, or what we would call an assistant matron, and in charge of quite a few hospital wards. He had a real way with patients. There was one particular lady, Mrs Mumford, who had head and neck cancer. As part of her surgery, she had a flap of skin taken from her breast to cover the spot where the cancer had been removed from under her chin. But together with that flap of skin from her breast came the nipple. Richard arrived one day, saw the nipple protruding from her chin and sat down on Mrs Mumford's bed.

'How about we just put a bandaid on that for you, Mrs Mumford.'

I was slowly beginning to understand that the patient always came first. During my consolidation, I was covering both the gynaecological and the head and neck wards when one lady in 'gynie' called me over. It was at the end of my shift, 12.30 pm– 9 pm, and I was saying goodnight to all the patients before I had to run down to South Kensington to catch the 9.30 pm Tube back to my flat in Ravenscourt Park. This woman had cervical cancer – stage 4 – and had run out of options.

'Keith, have you got a minute?' she asked, just before I was about to leave. Even though I had just a few minutes to make the Tube, I always made time for my patients. 'Sure thing,' I said. She took my hand and sat me down on the bed and looked deep into my eyes.

'Keith, am I dying?'

'Yes, you are,' I said, and I still remember her expression to this day. Her whole face lit up and a lot of the pain in her features seemed to be wiped away.

'Thank you,' she said, and I asked her why she was thanking me. 'Because no one has told me that before. Now I can let go, I can't fight anymore. But can you help me?'

'With what?' I asked.

'My husband, Peter,' she said. 'You've got to help me prepare him for my death.'

She was just 33 years old and only lived for nine more days, but after we spoke the change in her was remarkable. In the early days, we were taught to ask, 'What did the doctor say?' or 'How do you feel?' when asked this confronting question. But in my later training, particularly at the Marsden, it was decided honesty was the best policy. I was still only in my late 20s, and while I'd already faced some difficult and emotional periods with patients in their final days, this woman taught me a lot about death and dying. She taught me, as a young nurse doing my cancer training, how to die with dignity, and also a lot about being honest. She asked me a direct question, looked deep into my eyes, and before I knew it I was telling her the truth. I missed the 9.30 pm train that night.

In those days, medical staff were all about preserving life at all costs. But you've got to have a quality of life, and there's no use extending someone's life if they don't have that quality, so I gave her the permission she thought she needed to die, or perhaps it was that I helped her accept the inevitability of her situation. It wasn't about keeping someone alive, whatever the consequence; rather it was about the patient understanding and accepting the fact that they have terminal cancer and are going to die, and as a nurse, it was my job to help prepare them for that. So I decided that if a patient ever asked me that question again, I would be truthful with them.

Apart from always having the patients' best interests at heart, the Marsden staff also encouraged you to sit on the bed and hold the patient's hand to comfort them, whereas I had been trained with strict protocols whereby you were considered to be contaminating the bed if you sat on it. Back in Sydney, they didn't like you talking to patients either, as you were considered to be wasting time that would be better utilised cleaning bedpans or changing sheets. At the Marsden, we also used to go around before lunch and dinner with a drinks trolley, so patients could have a light ale, Guinness or sherry before meals, which was meant to stimulate their appetite. We went around later in the night, too, and rather than handing out sleeping tablets, we offered warm milk and a scotch or brandy.

When I got back to Royal Prince Alfred many months later, I tried to introduce some of those Marsden initiatives. 'No, no!' I was told. 'The nurses will be drinking all the alcohol.' But that never happened at the Marsden, as far as I knew. Later, although the RPA hospital administrators never knew it, I kept a bottle of scotch in the lower drawer of my office desk and I'd sometimes get it out if a patient or relative was very upset or they'd lost a loved one. The other thing that struck me about the Marsden was that we allowed patients to self-care. We would teach them to change their trachea tube or insert a nasal–gastric feed and it was these and other ideas about nursing that offered me a different perspective on patient care, removing the stricter guidelines and the almost military aspect of nursing that I was accustomed to. But I found it very difficult to continue with the Marsden way when I got home, so eventually I gave up. It would be some years before any of those practices that I picked up at the Marsden would be accepted in Australia.

9

RETURNING HOME

After spending nine fantastic months travelling around Europe in the orange Kombi and two years in London finishing my cancer training, I was offered a fulltime position at the Marsden. But the pay was poor, my parents still hadn't fully recovered from the injuries sustained in their home invasion, and despite them returning to the shop, the event had rocked them both. My friends Belinda and Barb were returning to Sydney, so I decided to head home, too, arriving in March 1981.

When I returned to RPA, Martin Tattersall and 'Rossie' McPherson had decided to create a position for me. I was to be an oncological supervisor. Apparently, it was all part of their grand plan. At the time, there were only three oncology units in Sydney, and despite having sworn I would never go back to RPA because I had already spent a decade there, I wanted to continue my work in cancer and there were only two other places in Sydney that specialised in cancer care.

So I settled for the devil I knew and returned to work at RPA.

At first, I worked on the relieving roster, before I was suddenly asked to take over as charge sister of Alfred block on Level 7 (A7). At the time, A7 was a large medical ward. The charge sister wasn't coping; she was on the verge of a nervous break-down and so distraught she could hardly complete her handover and left the next day, so I had scant details. The head of the unit, Dr John Greenaway, gave me several urgent jobs to do. The most pressing was to find another place for a notorious patient named Frank who had muscular dystrophy and was on a respi-rator. Only in his 20s, Frank was paralysed from the chest down, had no use of his arms or hands and had been on the wards for many months where he had been causing a few problems. Like all young men, Frank had physical needs, some of which we couldn't accommodate, and many nurses on the ward had been complaining about him. When they were washing him down he would get aroused and would indicate he'd like a bit more than a sponge down! The poor young female nurses, many in their late teens, didn't know how to handle it and it was soon brought to my attention, so I arranged to meet Frank's social worker.

'Between you and me,' the social worker said, 'I think I have a solution. Why don't we call in a lady of the night?'

Well, this solution was new to me, so I said, 'I'll leave it in your hands, so to speak.'

I only worked day shifts and wasn't on nights, and while I had discussed the proposition with senior staff, no one else knew our plans. So an escort arrived late one evening and dealt with Frank there and then. I'm not even sure how we paid her –

all the senior nurses probably did a whip-round! But after we sorted out Frank's physical needs, we still needed to resolve the overall Frank issue, so I decided to ring my friend Rob Kildy (my old 2IC at BP4) who was then in charge of Dame Eadith Walker Yaralla, a convalescent ward in Concord, which would better suit Frank rather than an acute ward.

'Before you say "no", Rob, I want to put something to you,' I said to her. 'How do you feel about having someone on a respirator in your ward? I'll have the gasman deliver a couple of large oxygen cylinders to you, if you are happy to keep him there.'

While I gave her as much medical information as I could, I downplayed the details about Frank's other needs, and after lots of planning, Frank was eventually dispatched to Yaralla, where his medical conditions could be better managed. John Greenaway was particularly thankful about Frank's move and while he never asked, I'm sure John had no idea what we had to do to address that patient's particular needs.

While I enjoyed returning to RPA to continue nursing, more difficult times lay ahead for my family. In the year I returned, Dad was injured again, this time working on the farm. He went to pump water to the chook sheds from the dam on the hill when he got in the way of one of the eight to ten sheep he ran. Dad was as light as a feather and a sheep easily knocked him over, breaking his collarbone as he fell, so it was back to Goulburn Base Hospital for my father, leaving Mum to run the business.

'I can't stay here by myself,' she said after Dad was admitted, so Brian took her home to Goulburn and they shut up shop again. We all decided, along with Mum, that we'd have to get Dad to sign over the power of attorney to Brian because there was no way they were going back to Cullerin and the shop. We cleared the house and put the property and the business on the market, and it sold soon after. Luckily for us, the sale went through just as rumours were emerging of a new highway bypassing Cullerin. That would signal the end of any traffic.

Meanwhile Fay – aka Sister Chrys – was still in WA working with Aboriginal communities but was keen to return home. 'We think you should go back to Goulburn,' she was told by her superiors. 'There's a position for you at the St John of God Hospital in Goulburn and your parents need you.'

So Fay headed home, and after a couple of months in Goulburn Base Hospital, Dad was transferred to St John of God Hospital where Fay could care for him. Mum lived in a little flat for a while before we sold the business and property at Cullerin. With the proceeds from the sale, we bought Mum a beautiful old colonial house in Goulburn. It was ideal because it had a big gate to a rear laneway that led into St John of God Hospital, so not only could Mum visit Dad but Fay could keep an eye on them both. Mum visited every day but Dad was slowly deteriorating, and after several months in hospital, he had a stroke.

'Keith, they don't think that your dad will live very long,' Mum said when she rang me. 'Do you want to come down?'

Because I had witnessed this slow decline before, and I had already said my goodbyes, I didn't want to see him like that again. William 'Bill' Cox died, aged 78, on 6 January 1982, almost three years after the bashing.

*

'What's for lunch?' Fay asked Mum one late winter afternoon in 1986. 'Oh, I feel like fish and chips,' Mum said, and Fay said, 'I do too.' So Fay went down to Auburn Street and returned with steaming fish and chips wrapped in white wax paper only to find Mum slouched in her chair. She had suffered a stroke but was still breathing. Fay called an ambulance, but rather than take Mum to Goulburn Base Hospital, Fay arranged for her to be admitted to St John of God next door. I arrived the next day along with all of Mum's other 'chickadees'.

'It will be a blessing when she goes,' Fay said when we arrived. Those who were able to come home stayed at Mum's house, including Coral who had followed Fay over to Western Australia. In the early hours of Monday morning, Coral took a phone call. 'It's the hospital, they've asked us to come,' she said. 'Mum's just had another stroke.'

As we walked the short distance to the hospital, Mum was taking her last breaths. Our dear Mum, Pansy, died on 7 July, aged 75, four and half years after Dad passed away. The nuns – colleagues of our sister Fay – treated us beautifully. They put us in a big room and gave us cups of tea and made Mum look nice. They lit a candle and in that light Pansy Cox (nee Dorsett) looked 20 years younger. All her wrinkles and her worries had faded away and everything was so peaceful as we gathered for a final farewell.

I've seen a lot of deaths in my five decades of nursing, some in terrible circumstances, but when it is personal, when it is family, it's very different. While you do use some of those coping mechanisms you acquire as a nurse, losing a parent or loved one is a lot harder than losing a patient.

10

KEITH AND THE CHEMETTES

By the early 1980s, the push was on at RPA to create a ward specifically for cancer patients. That first ward was created on Level 9 in E (Edinburgh) Block and I had some input as to what was required, not only from a ward perspective but also regarding what we wanted to have in a special unit where patients would be treated with chemotherapy. We ended up with a 30-bed ward just for cancer patients. Derek Raghavan had an office on the same floor, while Martin Tattersall was in the Blackburn Building where the Ludwig Institute was based. The institute was set up by American businessman Daniel K. Ludwig in 1971 to support cancer research and consists of an army of distinguished scientists dedicated to preventing and controlling cancer. While I was employed by RPA, my supervisor's salary was paid for by the Ludwig Institute, and cancer services at RPA were growing all the time with more chemotherapy and better cancer drugs. As a nurse, I was constantly learning new treatments – what cancers they were given for, the side effects, the drug's profile, how to administer it and if it was given singly or in a combination. The ever-changing nature of the treatment was one of the things I liked about cancer nursing. It wasn't mundane or routine. This informed my philosophy throughout my career – to always seek better ways to treat cancer and look after cancer patients – and it's why I later got involved in research. I always wanted to find ways to improve a patient's quality of life or adjust their treatment to make things easier for them. The changes I made might start as just a quality improvement, but then they might go on to form a pilot or research study.

For several years the chemotherapy nursing team at RPA – consisting of Alison Kirkby, Michele Carey and Kim Burke – was known as 'the Rovers' or 'Keith and the girls', and occasionally as 'KC and the Sunshine Band' – a sign of the times, no doubt. However, in the latter half of the 1980s, then-registrar Geoff Lindeman – now quite well known as Professor of Oncology at The Walter + Eliza Institute in Melbourne – coined the expression 'Keith and the Chemettes'. It was a label that stuck and over the years it became a name that many nurses wore with pride.

By 1986, I had become an oncology nurse consultant and was in charge of the chemotherapy team. In those years, up to 90 per cent of people with cancer were treated as inpatients. Some came in for symptom management, some for diagnosis, others because they were having a problem and some were having chemotherapy. Over the years, that trend has reversed, and only about 10 per cent of people who now have chemotherapy have it as an inpatient.

During this time, in an era of wide lapels, padded shoulders and long lunches, the nursing team had a memorable experience with the pharmaceutical representatives trying to sell drugs to the hospital. These reps were generally only interested in buttering up doctors because nurses could not order drugs. However, we nurses did have the ear of those who could. I must admit I had a way with people, and somehow I managed to persuade our local drug rep to take our team out for dinner. The choice was Alexandra's, a then rather swanky restaurant in Hunters Hill, and the pharmaceutical company would foot the bill. A night out at a fancy restaurant, paid for by someone else, was like an annual bonus for any nurse on a low wage. So the Chemettes, who by this time had grown in number, doubling in size, and including Tish Lancaster, went out for dinner. We put on our best dining-out finery, which for me included a cream linen jacket of which I was very fond.

My female colleagues had nicknamed the drug rep 'the Lizard', as it reflected how they felt about him. I was the only male nurse among many female nurses that night, but the drug rep brought along several of his rough-and-ready male colleagues who my female colleagues soon dubbed 'thugs in suits'. While we initially thought we'd pulled off the ultimate coup, we all quickly learned there's no such thing as a free lunch or, in this case, dinner. Lizard and his friends spent the whole night trying to feel up the Chemettes under the dining table, while a clumsy waiter spilt red wine all over my cream linen jacket – the highlight of my very stylish wardrobe at the time – and ruined it forever. One of the nurses, who had a glass or two, even managed to fall asleep at the table! The whole night out was pretty much a disaster for all the women at the table, while I managed to survive unscathed, apart from a wine-stained linen jacket. Needless to say, it was the first and last dinner we had with Lizard and his thuggish mates.

Every day, 'Keith and the Chemettes' went from ward to ward administering an array of drugs required to kill various cancers. We were ubiquitous throughout RPA because we had to administer the cytotoxic drugs across the length and breadth of the hospital before the dedicated ward for cancer patients came into being in 1986. Prior to that, we also held outpatient clinics Monday to Friday in Brown Street Outpatients which was accessed via the Page Chest Pavilion, then we took up residence on the whole ground floor of Gloucester House, or Gloucester 2, as it became known. We had a clinic and chemotherapy rooms, doctors' offices, and I had a nice office overlooking a big jacaranda in the courtyard. The clinics and chemotherapy unit were then relocated to Gloucester 5 floor, and my office was across from the chemotherapy pharmacy. Gloucester 6 was where all the offices for the medical staff and heads of departments for cancer services were located, and there was a conference room on that floor where all our meetings were held. But by that stage, we were bursting at the seams and Lifehouse was still many years away.

Space was at a premium and we used the Special Unit on Level 9 of E Block, which had just two beds and three chairs, for the administration of chemotherapy treatment as an outpatient, and also administered chemo at Brown Street Outpatients. In those days, with a lack of awareness around work health and safety, these toxic drugs were prepared under a perspex hood with little ventilation. We used gloves and material gowns but not the protective Tyvek suits which were used later, or the distinctive purple gowns and nitrile gloves in use today. So through the 1970s and 1980s, these drugs were mixed and administered by many hundreds of nurses. They are highly toxic chemical treatments that kill not only cancer cells but normal cells, including red and white blood cells and platelets. Because of this, female staff handling those drugs were discouraged from falling pregnant as the drugs were also known to cause birth defects. Back then personal protective equipment (PPE) and protection from occupational hazards also weren't at the level that is required now, and clinical nursing staff were commonly exposed to cytotoxic drugs, especially during the administration and disposal of medicines. It was risky. Despite the pregnancy warnings, six female nurses who did fall pregnant miscarried or had babies with abnormalities which ranged from harelip and cleft palate to a hole in the heart, webbed fingers or spinal abnormalities. In a small team, that is quite a high number. Sadly, several of the Chemettes were also diagnosed with breast cancer and it has claimed the lives of two nurses who I worked with and knew well. Two other nursing colleagues were also diagnosed with breast cancer but have survived, including one who was later treated at Chris O'Brien Lifehouse.

At one stage in the late 1980s, blood tests and urine samples were taken from RPA nurses who were administering the drugs, with the tests monitored by Flinders Medical Centre in Adelaide. It was discovered that one of our RPA chemotherapy nurses, who had prepared a substantial amount of the cytotoxic drugs, had mutagens in her urine. This was the same nurse who was diagnosed with breast cancer three decades later. This was also the nurse who had the longest exposure to the drugs, as she had been a chemotherapy nurse mixing and administering the same drugs at the Royal Marsden Hospital, London, in the 1970s, who I knew from my early days at RPA.

At present, there is no proven link to breast cancer in the use or administration of cytotoxic drugs, but I am convinced it has affected my own health. While I administered cytotoxins, my platelet count was never above 100,000 per microlitre while the average person's count is about 150,000–400,000 per micro-litre. I was always getting cold sores and mouth ulcers and my immune system was quite poor. At one stage, I was even sent to see an immunologist. I was a redhead back then and had a full head of hair, and while we redheads generally have a lower platelet count, they never credited mine to the chemo drugs I was handling. The immunologist put me on a carrot a day to boost my carotene, and it also helps with the mucosal lining in the mouth, but you can't have too much carrot in your diet, as your palms go yellow and too much carotene blocks the hepatic system or common bile duct.

But nurses are no longer involved in the mixing of the cyto-toxic drugs in hospital wards as pharmacy departments took over their preparation in the early 1990s. They now use modern machinery and techniques including isolators and laminar-flow hoods to protect them, and the work is done off-site. Today, anyone – male or female – who intends to have a baby in the near future is strongly discouraged from working in chemo-therapy as there continues to be a high risk of birth defects from any contact with cancer-killing drugs.

★

Despite the seriousness of our business, oncologist Dr Derek Raghavan was one of those good-natured people who instigated many social activities outside of work, and he was involved in all of our social activities on the wards, too. Morale was pretty good overall, and distractions such as our cake-making competition and car rallies, which I helped organise, would boost spirits. We also had a cocktail-making competition which involved everyone gathering at E9 Special Unit on a Friday afternoon, after most of our work was done. It was the early 1990s, and E9 Special Unit was a separate space for outpatients in between two wards at the end of a corridor, so we pretty much had it to ourselves at the end of the week. And being at the end of a long week – long before random breath testing was introduced – it was also a good spot to relax with a few staff drinks.

Each Friday after work, I would ask for volunteers and they'd pair up or I'd pair people up and they'd have to come back to the ward the following Friday with a cocktail concoction, connected somehow to work we were doing in cancer care. Like the cake competition, you had to put in a big effort in the presentation of your concoction and tell people what the story was behind it. One week, Derek and Robin Stuart-Harris, now Emeritus Professor at ANU, decided to create a version of the new cancer drug cocktail, methotrexate and 5-FU, also known as fluorouracil. Methotrexate is a yellow colour and fluoro-uracil is clear, so they decided to deconstruct the combination by draining all the saline out of a Solupak bag and loading it with orange juice, and then connecting that to a clear fluid – aka 5-FU – which they had replaced with vodka. Dressed in tuxedos, bow ties and each wearing Spider-Man masks – don't ask me why – they proceeded to 'administer' the cocktail by turning on the roller clamp on the Solupak which would then mix the orange juice with the vodka.

Many staff went to a lot of trouble to impress and it was quite an expensive process as you had to make enough cocktails for 30 or 40 people. One year, my Chemette colleague Michele Carey and I took out the annual award for best cocktail with what we called 'the 101', as we figured we had made that many ourselves over the several years that the competition had been in place. We presented the 101s on a silver tray, with me in a hired bright red shirt and toreador jacket and pants and Michele in a matching red flamenco dress. Our 101 had all sorts of liqueurs and spirits in it and was finished off with cream, as was the fashion at the time, and we had people ringing up for weeks afterwards, asking for the recipe, which, in case you were wondering, is this:

The 101
> 8 ice cubes
> ⅓ of a cocktail shaker of orange juice
> 2 nips Galliano
> 2 nips Grand Marnier
> 2 nips Drambuie
> 20 millilitres cream
> *Makes 4–6. Garnish with orange and glacé cherries and don't drive home afterwards.*

★

Weekends meant more time to relax and this was where our car rallies began. Introduced by Derek, he and his wife Trish and two daughters would map out a particular route and we would have to end up at a particular destination, usually about two hours later, having taken care to note all the clues and turn at all of the correct spots along the way. At the end, we'd eat, have a few drinks, and the winner would be presented with a trophy made from an old hubcap.

The car rallies always started on a Sunday outside RPA and on one particular weekend, longstanding oncology professor and statistician Alan Coates was taking part. In addition to treating breast cancer patients, which was his specialty, he also compiled vast amounts of statistics from clinical cancer trials to use in further studies, medical research papers and clinical papers. One of the early clues at this rally was to head to a nearby roundabout and make a 360-degree turn, then go back the way you'd come. But Alan did a 180 and kept on going in the wrong direction. As a numbers man, he should have known better. There was an envelope to open in the event of emergencies, giving the final destination. Alan was forced to open the letter and eventually turned up two hours after everyone else. He has since survived three cardiac arrests, with the keen church bell-ringer once winched to safety from the belltower of St Mary's Cathedral. So his number is not up just yet.

While I presume there is still some camaraderie on the wards, sadly, I'm sure none of these activities takes place now, with more work for nurses, fewer resources and greater responsibility heaped upon our healthcare workers.

11

A STATESMAN TO ORANGE

HEIDI STEWART (1971–1993)

While I get on extremely well with young people, I do find it harder to care for children with cancer because when they die, they haven't lived a life. Someone like me has had the chance to enjoy my life, a very full life, and while I don't particularly want to die, I've had a great time and done a lot of things. But a young person who is in high school, or doing their HSC year, who is making new lifelong friends, who loves sport, has just started their journey: they haven't really lived.

By the time I met Heidi Stewart in June 1992, she had already been diagnosed with sarcoma and undergone surgery to remove part of her leg, and the cancer had spread to her lungs. She was a very intelligent girl and also very determined. Even during her treatment, Heidi continued to attend uni as, influenced by her illness, she wanted to pursue a career in medicine. As her parents lived in Orange in rural NSW and she was at

Sydney University, she chose to live in The Women's College, which was conveniently just down the road from both the hospital and the university.

Martin Tattersall and I were very fond of Heidi. She was special: effervescent, oozing personality, and everyone liked her. Despite her partial amputation, she was confident in herself and didn't let the loss of one leg deter her from getting on with things. She would have made a brilliant doctor. The duration of her illness was a lot longer than many other patients who I had seen over the years. Heidi had round after round of chemotherapy and radiotherapy over about 18 months. But her illness continued to progress.

One day I went up to 10 South – the same ward where Chris O'Brien would later spend his last hours – and Heidi was with Norelle Lickiss, her palliative care physician. We needed to discuss her current condition, so Narelle, Martin and I went into the room with Heidi and her father, Ian, who'd come down from Orange. We told them that Heidi's time was short and there was not a lot we could do for her, apart from managing her symptoms. I thought it was all we had to offer. Heidi was still conscious and alert and accepted what we had told her.

'I want to go home. I don't want to die here. I want to die at home,' she said. It was not a plea, just a request, and not an unusual one for someone in her condition. But achieving it would prove to be challenging, and the way we went about it would probably not be allowed today. We all talked about the logistics and then I said to Heidi, 'Leave it with me.' Martin, Narelle and I went into the clinical room and we were all quite upset. We weren't blubbering, as you have to keep your composure, but it's the first time I'd ever seen Martin Tattersall cry.

He was a stoic Yorkshireman, very matter-of-fact, and rarely if ever revealed his emotions in front of staff or even behind closed doors as far as I knew.

'Are you all right, Prof?' I asked.

'If I had a daughter, I would have liked her to be just like Heidi,' he said.

Heidi was not well enough to fly, and while she could go by road ambulance, that would also be difficult. We could tell by looking at Heidi — and I was fairly experienced by then — that she was not going to live very long. By that stage she had metastatic disease, meaning her cancer had spread; she had limited lung capacity and was in a lot of pain. But we got on with the job and talked about how we could take her back to Orange.

'I want to drive her home,' her father said, not perturbed by the fact that Orange was a 250-kilometre, three-and-a-half-hour drive away. He just wanted to fulfil his daughter's last wish.

'You can't drive her home by yourself,' I said, and then I told Narelle and Prof that I'd see what I could do. I rang my boss, told her the story, and she gave the OK for me to accompany them. While things were a lot more flexible in those days, it still took 24 hours for the hospital to give me official permission and to organise the pain relief we needed for Heidi's trip home. I also had to arrange colleagues in Bathurst to be an emergency backup along the way, and nursing care for Heidi after she arrived home in Orange. The family wouldn't be able to manage all her palliative care by themselves and I wasn't going to just leave her there.

We were scheduled to leave RPA around lunchtime and were due to arrive in Orange in the early evening, about 4–5 pm. The hospital was able to give me what I thought would be enough morphine, syringes, oxygen and all the other supplies we would need for the road trip. Heidi's father's car was a two-tone, brown-and-cream Holden Statesman, quite a large and comfortable car and perfect for long drives in the country, but it was no ambulance. We laid the front passenger seat down completely with Heidi lying almost flat with the seatbelt across her waist. I sat in the back of the car, behind Heidi, so I could keep checking on her condition. And so, preparations finally complete, we set off.

We stopped several times on the side of the road along the way as I could neither draw up the morphine from the vial while we were driving along, nor attempt to administer Heidi's pain relief on the move. Today they use a syringe driver, a drug-loaded machine which almost does the job for you, whereas in those days you had to give a subcutaneous injection with what we call a butterfly needle into a muscle. By the time we'd got over the mountains and were coming into Bathurst, I'd run out of morphine. With all the bumpy, windy roads and corners and weaving of the car, more morphine was required to keep Heidi pain-free than I had realised. I'd also used up some spare vials meant for her care at home. No more morphine meant a stop at Bathurst Hospital a bit further on. I'd trained a lot of the cancer nurses in Bathurst – and Orange and Dubbo, for that matter – so I knew a few of them who had come to RPA over the years.

I rang Barbara Wren, the nurse in charge of the oncology unit in Bathurst, and told her what I needed. I wasn't a nurse practitioner at that stage, so I couldn't prescribe drugs myself and neither could Barbara, so we had to organise a doctor to do so. We left Heidi in the car with her father because it was too hard to get her in and out. Barb did a great job in quickly getting what we needed, and we gave Heidi some more morphine on the spot and took enough to get us to Orange. We arrived there about 45 minutes after we left Bathurst, the end of a very long and fraught four-hour haul, but we made it. I might have said a few prayers on the way, too.

The family lived on a beautiful property, 'Hei-Mel', in a lovely old house outside of town and all of Heidi's family, most of whom I had met during her treatment, were there to meet us. We got Heidi out of the car, took her into her room and made her as comfortable as we could. We arrived around 5 pm and the community nurses had finished for the day, so I taught the family how to administer Heidi's pain relief, with her mother, Sue, and older sister, Melinda, taking on the main roles as carers. I had dinner with the family while Heidi slept, exhausted by the long trip.

I didn't sleep very much that night as I was listening out for her. Although her family were ever-present, I was pretty much the nurse on call, and I got up a couple of times during the night to check on her. The next morning we had breakfast and everyone felt comfortable enough to be able to take over Heidi's care. She was semi-conscious, and mostly slept, but I went in and said goodbye. It was a very hard thing to do but I managed to keep it all together.

The family had made arrangements to put me on a flight to Sydney that morning, and as I got back into the Statesman with Heidi's father, Melinda came running out clutching a photo in a frame. It was a picture of Heidi and her younger sister Anna, 15 at the time, on the back of a boat. The photo was of the Stewarts' last family holiday to Treasure Island in Fiji.

'Heidi would like you to have this photo,' said Melinda as she passed it through the driver's side window. Her dad started crying, then I started crying, and we both cried all the way to the airport.

Heidi died on 18 December 1993, 18 days after the trip in the Statesman. She was first diagnosed in March 1989, when she was in Year 12, and lived for four years and nine months after that. Heidi could have chemo in the morning and complete an exam in the afternoon and still gain a distinction. She eventually received a Bachelor of Arts, was mentioned in the honour roll in the *Sydney Morning Herald* for her results and was accepted into Medicine at Sydney University.

It is hard to put into words, but some patients have more of an impact on you than others. While you meet many people throughout your life, not all of them become close friends. It's the same with patients, some you emotionally connect with more than others. Heidi's intellect and beautiful personality left an impression on the lives of many and that includes me to this day.

12

CANTEEN VIA CONCORDE

I have always found working with young people to be meaningful, which is why in the 1990s I became involved in CanTeen,
which is an organisation for adolescent cancer patients and their
families. Teenage patients didn't go into a paediatric hospital
unless they were under 15, and if they were older they went into
an adult hospital where the patient in the next bed could be
80 or 90 years old. The needs of adolescents are different from
those of adults, but also different from the needs of children.
I felt there was a big gap in the system and was quite passionate
about it, so I became a volunteer for CanTeen and remained so
for 25 years.

In 1997, early on in the piece, CanTeen had raised enough
money, with the help of donations from Qantas and British
Airways, to take five 'CanTeenians' to the USA and on to the
UK via Concorde. Another nurse was supposed to be accompanying them on the trip, but had to pull out. With just a week or

so to go, the organisers were looking for a male nurse replace-ment to accompany the kids on the trip, and as I was already involved with CanTeen, I was approached to be their chaper-one. I went to see my boss, told her what they wanted me to do and asked if I could have a two-week holiday. 'Yes,' she said. 'You're doing great work.'

The youngest on this global tour was James, a 13-year-old from Nowra who was the sibling of a cancer patient. Then there was Emma, 16, who had thyroid cancer and was in remission. Adam was the eldest, about 21 or 22 at the time, and he had leukaemia and was on maintenance chemotherapy. Kim, 15, had a sarcoma, and she'd already had one leg amputated below the knee. Then there was another young fellow, Paul, 17, who had a form of leukaemia. He'd finished his treatment but had remaining side effects from his chemotherapy, which included osteoporosis, or weakening of the bone, and he was on calliper crutches. While it was to be a whirlwind tour – circumnavigating the globe in 15 days, visiting Las Vegas, New York, then flying to London via Concorde and on to Singapore before heading home – I had to be a chaperone and pseudo parent as well as a nurse, making sure they were all cared for and that they took their medi-cation. It was a big responsibility, and as exciting as it was to think about jumping on the Concorde in New York and arriving a few hours later in London, it was daunting. I didn't have much time to prepare, either, as I got the call-up very late and I didn't meet the kids or their parents until just before we left. In fact, it was the night before we departed when I met each of the parents at the Travelodge in Camperdown, just down the road from RPA.

'Keith, so and so needs his medication at this time', and 'So and so has to have this done', and 'Our girl has to be in bed at this time'. The parents were naturally a bit nervous about releasing their charges into my care for their first big trip away from home, but it meant I not only had all the kids to look after but their parents' expectations to manage as well. *God*, I thought, *what have I let myself in for?*

When we took off the next day, I was also the de facto travel guide. I had to collect the kids' passports, check them all in along with their luggage, get them through Customs, and all the other stuff that goes with international travel. We flew from Sydney to Los Angeles, a long flight by anyone's standards. Once in LA we headed to Anaheim and on to Disneyland. Kim decided to try her prosthesis despite the prospect of walking around Disneyland for hours on end. Paul also said he would be all right, even though he'd have to support his weight on calliper crutches all day. Well, in the end, they couldn't manage, as it was a long day and Disneyland is vast. Kim ended up with blisters on her stump and Paul was also exhausted by the end of day one of our two-day visit, so we organised two wheelchairs for the second day. That was quite helpful in the end, as there were a lot of long queues to get on the rides, but because our group had two people in wheelchairs, we were all allowed into the priority queue. Adam, James, Emma and I would take turns pushing the wheelchairs. After that, I insisted on Paul and Kim using wheelchairs for our big outings.

After Disneyland, we went to Las Vegas – not a great place to take kids, as we couldn't go into any of the casinos, but the buildings were amazing. From there we went to Pittsburgh, where we were greeted by the mayor and made to feel very special. The city invited us to the Crayola factory, which was quite fascinating. We then visited the police station, where they 'arrested' James and frightened the life out of him. We also went to Larry Holmes's boxing studio where we met the man himself and he signed autographs for everyone. I am not really into boxing, but it was very kind of him and the kids loved it. From Pittsburgh we were chauffeured to New York, where we visited the Australian Consulate and met the staff. Andrew Peacock was the Australian Ambassador at the time but he was away at an Anzac Day event, so while we didn't get to meet him, I have a picture of me sitting in his chair.

New York was one of the most memorable stops on our trip because, as we were guests of the Australian Consulate, they organised everything from a helicopter ride around Manhattan to tickets to the Broadway show *Tap Dogs*, which featured an all-Australian cast. We also had a backstage tour where we met the cast, a real highlight. We had a tour of the New York Police Department headquarters where we dressed up in riot gear – a helmet, heavy vest and guns – fortunately, unloaded. Wherever we went, we were showered with attention – except for our hotel, where hygiene didn't seem a priority. But that's another story! After two days in New York, we boarded our Concorde flight at LaGuardia Airport and were due to arrive at Heathrow three hours and twenty minutes later.

Concorde seated 100 passengers and was divided into two sections, with 40 seats at the front, a service area in the middle and 60 seats to the rear. The seats were two-by-two with a narrow aisle in the middle and not much headroom. We departed on time and settled in for a meal, served on Royal Doulton crockery, eaten with Christofle silver cutlery, and drinks were poured into Waterford Crystal glassware. After we ate, a flight attendant approached James after she noticed him starting to wrap up all the Christofle, Royal Doulton and Waterford.

'What are you doing?' she said.

'I hope you don't mind,' James responded, 'but I'd like to take this home to my mother.'

'Don't do that!' she said. 'They're all dirty. I'll give you a clean set.'

I'm sure there is now a lovely set of Concorde cutlery sitting in a side table in a dining room somewhere in Nowra.

On top of that, we were all given a tour of the tiny flight deck, and when I got back to my seat I found two bottles of wine waiting – an expensive red and a French champagne. We were also given a leather attaché case, which came with a subtly branded leather chequebook holder and silver pen, all of which I still have today. But the trip to London went all too quickly, and I wanted to go back to New York and start all over again.

Because we were returning to the airport for our activities the next day, we were billeted out to various families near Heathrow for the night. Back at the airport in the morning, I got to fly a Jumbo. It was in fact a simulator, but I was able to revisit our Heathrow landing from the day before. To pass the exam, you had to take off and land in wet as well as dry weather, plus land and take off at night, and during the day, and in a heavy fog. Taking off was not as hard as landing and you had to keep the crosshairs on the stability gauge even. I even had to abort once. 'Keith, you're going a bit to the left,' the captain said, and it felt like I really was in the plane. But I didn't crash and I passed the test with flying colours. All the kids had a go, too, and received their certificates, as did I.

After our simulator experience, we checked into our London hotel and the following day started a full itinerary which had been organised by the local Lions Club. It included Buckingham

Palace, the Tower of London and various other highlights. Later that afternoon, we all gathered in the boys' room. We were nearing the end of our 15-day tour and everyone was exhausted. The kids said they just wanted a day off, to do some shopping, get some souvenirs and just have a look around. I'd lived in London before and had been back several times since, so I knew it well and was able to take the kids up to Oxford Street where they could buy their own trendy Dr Martens boots and a bunch of souvenirs for family and friends. But that's where we lost James. We were in a group and had all left this one shop, or at least I thought we had, but he was still in there. I thought he'd followed us, but after we were a fair way down the street, I said: 'Where's James?' No one knew, so I said, 'Look, you all stay here and I'll backtrack.'

I was panicking because it was Oxford Street, just about the busiest place you could be in London, and there were so many people about. How do you tell a parent that you've taken their child overseas and then lost them? Thank goodness James had the sense to stay outside the same shop we'd been in, where I found him a few minutes later.

While we were able to find James, Adam was the one who worried me the most because he was having maintenance chemotherapy. He was in remission, but his medication was intended to stop a recurrence of his leukaemia. We flew business class from London, but by the time we got to Singapore, Adam was not well at all and had fevers. I even thought we might need to get his blood count checked. When we arrived at Changi Airport, we were greeted by the consular staff and taken to our hotel. I thought I'd be taking Adam to the hospital, but with some nursing care and help from the Australian Consulate, we avoided that. While Adam loved the trip the majority of the time, by then the poor boy just wanted to get home. The other kids were worn out too, as was I. The following day, I told the consular staff we'd regretfully have to cancel some of the itinerary, and we did as little as possible before boarding our flight home.

On the whole, however, that trip was an amazing experience. Opportunities like that don't arise very often, especially from a nurse or carer's perspective. You're often in the hospital, and that's your sole environment. But a trip like that can change everyone's perspective; it can allow kids to have a positive attitude and to enjoy life a bit more and not focus on their illness. The flight back to Sydney was the last leg of a very long and full itinerary. One of Qantas staffers said to me: 'Keith, you have a sleep, and if one of the kids has a problem we'll wake you up, otherwise we'll look after them.'

So I slept.

13

DROPPED BALLS, DRUGS AND HITLER

In the 1970s, young patients with testicular cancer usually died, simple as that. It was mainly because we didn't have good enough chemotherapy drugs and the cancer usually wasn't detected early enough, so by the time we knew about it, it was often too late.

The most common cause of testicular cancer is likely to be from an undescended testis at birth, known as cryptorchidism. During gestation, testes initially develop in the abdomen then, about a month before birth, they should drop down through the inguinal canal into the scrotum where they then adhere. But some men have undescended testes, where either one or both do not drop down. This occurs in about 5 per cent of males and about 30 per cent of baby boys born prematurely. It is one of the main risk factors for testicular cancer, and has often been the case for patients who are later diagnosed with the disease. Today orchiopexy, the operation to repair undescended testes, is usually conducted early in an infant's life. In this minor operation, the testes are pulled down through the inguinal canal then adhered or stitched to the scrotum. After that, the testes can maintain the correct environment and drop down when it is hot or draw up into the top part of the scrotum when it is cold. But if the testes do not descend into the scrotum and stay in the abdomen, testicular cancer may develop and can spread rapidly once it does. Other modes of spread may be via the inguinal canal or along the para-aortic lymph nodes which run along the main blood vessel, the aorta, which means that type of cancer has a fairly direct path to all the vital internal organs, potentially spreading to a patient's abdomen, liver, lungs and lymphatic nodes, then ultimately to the brain.

Today, cancer of the testes is one of the most common forms of cancer in men aged 15–32, and most predominantly among those aged 17–24, young men who have yet to live a full life. The reason I always had a passion for this group of patients is that they are young, their masculinity is still evolving and they need a very thorough, coordinated plan to take them through the treatment process. This was one area where I knew I could make an impact.

While breast cancer does affect some men, it is a particularly female-focused disease and has gained significant coverage in the media with great work by the McGrath Foundation and their specialised breast cancer nurses, among others. If you surveyed 100 men today in that at-risk age group and asked them: 'Have you heard about testicular cancer?' the majority would say 'Yes', but if you then asked them: 'Do you examine your testes once a month?' the majority would say 'No'. Despite testicular cancer and prostate cancer being the two main cancers in men, you hardly see the issue mentioned in the media, and rarely do you see diagrams showing men how to self-check as we do with breast cancer screening. If we could raise the profile of testicular cancer and get the subject into women's magazines – so girlfriends or wives would talk about it and maybe even check their partners themselves – then I'm sure that would help, but men need to take action too. The thing men need to ask themselves – or their partner – is, what is normal? With breast cancer, a woman needs to know what's normal for her breasts. Not everyone's the same: some women have very lumpy breasts, some get lumps at certain points in their menstrual cycle, so they need to know if that is normal for them. It's the same for men – they need to know what to check for. A lump could be a blood vessel, the epididymis, for example, which is the vessel that carries the sperm and semen and runs to the back of the testes, or the lump could have other causes.

As a male nurse, I felt I could bring a degree of comfort and familiarity into the delicate conversations we often needed to have with testicular cancer patients. I always tried to build a rapport with them, so that they felt OK talking to me about anything: their ups and downs, their fears, even their testicles. It's confronting for a patient to discuss their sexuality, sexual function, their relationships and so on. When they do, it's quite sensitive, and I liked to think they could feel confident discussing these things with me. Often we would end up forming a very close relationship. I feel very honoured and privileged to have been part of that.

Encouragingly, survival rates for testicular cancer have changed dramatically since the 1970s, and the reason why is threefold: first is the discovery and development of cisplatin, a platinum-based drug that kills cancer cells; second is early detection through better scanning, and third is a greater general awareness of testicular cancer.

Cisplatin, while a very effective drug, has several severe side effects, the main ones being nausea and vomiting. Where once we had to bring patients into hospital to treat them for both cancer and the nausea the treatment causes, over time and with the development of better anti-sickness medication, known as antiemetics, to counter those side effects, cisplatin has come into its own as a treatment for testicular cancer as well as many other cancers.

Also, as we know, men generally don't like to talk about illness and don't regularly perform self-examination, so any symptoms such as lumps often go unnoticed or unreported to a GP. A family history of undescended testes can be an indicator. As mentioned, testicular cancer may spread rapidly from a primary site to other sites unless you get on top of it early. However, with the evolution of new scans and ultra-sounds, and an improvement in rates of self-examination and awareness, there has been a rise in early detection. Not only that, attention has been drawn to the issue by people such as cyclist Lance Armstrong, who overcame a well-publicised battle with testicular cancer long before he was disgraced for using performance-enhancing drugs.

Today, through early detection, more effective treatment and better anti-sickness drugs, the percentage of those who survive testicular cancer is in the mid-90s. As with all cancers, there are a variety of cell types, some of which spread more rapidly than others, or have a higher malignancy than others. Take seminoma, for example. It is not quite as severe as other cancers and is, therefore, one of the most treatable and curable cancers around, with a survival rate above 95 per cent, if discovered in the early stages. Occurring in older males, it is usually treated by the removal of the affected testis, in addition to radiotherapy to the nodes. But on the other end of the scale is choriocarcinoma, the rarest and most aggressive form of testicular cancer, which has the potential to spread rapidly throughout the body including to the brain. When I started dealing with mostly young men with testicular cancer, part of the coordinated plan for treatment was to organise their blood tests, or 'bloods'. The bloods look for two particular tumour markers called alpha-fetoprotein and beta hCG. If these markers are not showing, then it is likely the cancer is a seminoma, but if the markers are extremely high, then you are probably looking at choriocarcinoma. If that was the case, further investigation was required.

Any cancer patient who is about to undergo chemotherapy, or in some cases radiotherapy, also needs to think quickly about fertility, as these treatments can render them infertile. In the case of males, sperm banking is strongly suggested, as many testicular cancer patients are in their adolescence or are young adults. They haven't even thought about what the future may hold for them – let alone having children. For a lot of these young men, their fertility does return to normal, but if it doesn't, a coordinated plan means they've got material in the bank, just in case. It always gave me great joy to be introduced to a former patient's first child down the track, knowing that I helped them on the path to fatherhood, despite their diagnosis.

In the very early days, we didn't have any testes prostheses either, and a lot of young men indicated that they would feel inadequate if they had to lose a testicle. Some older readers may recall a British World War II ditty, 'Hitler Has Only Got One Ball', which mocked the Nazi leader for having one testicle. This was deemed a good enough reason to question his manhood. As late as 2015, it was reported that Hitler's secret medical records revealed he had, in fact, one undescended testis. Patients used to say to me, 'But I'm now only half a man', so part of my job was helping them process a lot of that anxiety about sexuality and sexual function. Because having a testis removed doesn't mean they're infertile, can't have erections, have normal intercourse, ejaculate or maintain normal sexual function. Today, if a testis has been removed by a urologist, many patients have a prosthesis put in, but those prostheses still don't have quite the same profile as, say, breast implants. For me, being a male, I could not only relate to these patients but could easily talk to them about their sexuality and sexual function, as well as discuss fertility, sperm banking options and the side effects of chemotherapy.

In the late 1990s, I looked after eight young men on chemotherapy treatment for testicular cancer. Some of them were still in high school and most didn't even know what testicular cancer was before their diagnoses. Unlike self-examination for the detection of breast cancer, self-examination of the testes wasn't widely spoken about, and the mothers of some of these young men would say to me: 'We need to do something about this! We need to introduce the teaching of self-examination into schools.'

So several very passionate mothers were the driving force behind producing a fun video and brochure on self-examination aimed at teenagers and young men. On the front of the brochure was a picture of a chimpanzee swinging through the trees, hand covering its genitals, with the words, *Monkeys do it, so why not you?*

The accompanying video showed a technique by which young men could examine their testes once a month. The program, supported by Michael Boyer and myself, was promoted in schools throughout the Sydney metropolitan area and was very successful, leading to a greater number of early testicular cancer diagnoses. So mums and dads of young men, encourage your boys to check their balls!

CHARLES HAGENBACH (1964–2019)

Charles must have been in his 20s when I met him in the 1980s. He had moved from his family farm in Wagga Wagga, NSW, to WA to become a helicopter pilot and was working north of Perth when he became concerned by his scrotum, which had become enlarged. He didn't think much of it at the time, as he had been kicked by a sheep on the farm some months earlier. But the continued swelling of his testes prompted Charles to visit a doctor who immediately sent him to Perth, where he was diagnosed with a testicular mass that would need urgent treatment.

Because Charles didn't have any relatives in WA and few friends there, he wanted to return to NSW for treatment. Charles's doctor in Perth contacted Professor Derek Raghavan, an expert in genitourinary cancers, who was able to organise Charles's admission to RPA soon after his arrival on a commercial flight from WA. It was a Monday evening and while Derek couldn't meet Charles when he walked through the door, Michael Boyer stepped in. Michael was doing his oncology training at the time and took Charles's medical history and organised his blood tests. The next morning, X-rays and an ultrasound were taken and the results revealed that the cancer had spread from his testis to his chest. A CT scan also identified that the cancer had spread to the para-aortic lymph nodes.

The following day, after the diagnosis had been made, both Derek and Michael came to my door in the oncology ward on E9 North and asked if I could see a new patient. After telling me a little of Charles's history, Derek introduced us and we all went through the outline of the disease and the recommended treatment which would need to be rapid and systemic. It would start with chemotherapy to try to reduce the mass in his lungs and para-aortic lymph nodes and, hopefully, it would reduce the testicular mass as well. The usual procedure is to remove the infected testis and that remained a secondary option. John Rogers, a urologist, was called in, and he agreed with Derek's diagnosis. I was asked to go through the treatment with Charles and warn him of the side effects, which were still quite severe then as we didn't have the anti-sickness medication we do today. I'd also have to talk to him about his fertility as he was young, single and had no children. But, in the end, we didn't have enough time for sperm banking as his chemotherapy treatment needed to start immediately, even though it may have rendered him infertile.

Later that day, Charles's sister Emma and her fiancé Gary arrived at RPA, as they lived close by and, soon after, Charles's mother came up from Wagga Wagga. His father arrived a day after that, as did his brother Jeremy and sisters Tracey and Marie, so he had lots of family popping in and out and there was always a lot of action happening around his room. But I had to make sure he fully understood the chemotherapy and its potential side effects, which could include hearing loss from the cisplatin and impaired lung capacity from a drug called bleomycin.

Because of the urgency of Charles's situation, we started treatment pretty much straight away, and while he did suffer some side effects, overall he responded well. By the start of the following week, Charles was ready to be discharged and would live at his sister's house so he could return to RPA to continue his round of bleomycin treatment. In those days, we also gave the platinum treatment on day 1 of his 21-day treatment cycle, but because we didn't have the anti-sickness medicine that now exists, people became very ill, constantly vomiting, and we would need to keep a close eye on him. The cycle also included vinblastine on days 1 and 2 and bleomycin on days 1, 8 and 15.

Later, Charles underwent surgery too. John Rogers removed the cancerous testis, and then renowned cardiothoracic surgeon Brian McCaughan 'cherry-picked' what remained of the lesions on both of Charles's lungs and sent the samples off to pathology to see if there were any live cells left or whether the chemo had killed them all. But there was residual disease, so John had to perform a para-aortic lymph node dissection, opening Charles's abdomen from the belly button up, then stripping out all the nodes from both sides of the aorta. The risks associated with this type of surgery include chylous ascites, where there is a build-up of fluid in the abdomen, and if that doesn't drain, the 'chyle' takes a lot of protein from the body and a drip is required. By this time Charles had run out of veins and we had to put in a Hickman's line, a long hollow tube inserted into a vein in the chest and ending in a larger vein just above the heart, to get fluids into him. There were further complications over a period of eight months or so, but Charles overcame them all and never once complained, always remaining positive and cheerful.

His reward was that he eventually went into remission, and that continued for several years.

I got to know the family quite well over those intense months and the years that followed, so much so that Charles's sister Emma invited me to her wedding which was back on the family protea farm, Karrindee, near Uranquinty in the NSW Riverina. Charles was already back on the farm by then, but when he did return to Sydney for treatment or check-ups, he would arrive with huge bunches of beautiful proteas and my house would end up being full of them.

Emma and Gary's wedding ceremony was held on a big rock in the middle of a paddock with the sun setting in the background and it was a glorious sight. The reception was held on the family farm with the barn perfectly decorated with lots of proteas among the sparkling lights. I sat next to TV presenter Alex Wileman and we had a lovely chat. Overall, it was a memorable evening. It was made even better when, sometime later, Charles told me that he too was to marry, and Brian McCaughan, my nursing colleague Tish Lancaster – one of the early Chemettes – and I were all invited to the ceremony in Crookwell, just up the road from where I was brought up. A few years later Charles and Jane welcomed their first daughter into the world, then a few years after that a second, and later Charles had a son with a new partner, so despite all that he went through and all of his treatments and setbacks, he was still able to have children.

I continued to maintain contact with the family, which included visits to the farm and their beautiful homestead, but unfortunately, many years later, Charles relapsed. While it is not common, he did have what's called a mature teratoma and we started treatment again. Charles responded well, initially, and was again disease-free for a few years. But a second relapse revealed that the cancer had transformed and it took a few pathologists to work out what was going on before we tried further chemotherapy and radiotherapy. Charles had further surgery to remove a tumour in his brain and later had one of his scapula removed as the cancer was in his bones. All the while, Charles continued to be upbeat and didn't waste energy complaining.

By the time of his last relapse, cancer care at RPA had moved to Lifehouse and Charles was well impressed by the new offering and the way treatment had changed for the better in the intervening years. He had battled cancer for over three decades and seen the inside of E9, Gloucester House and Lifehouse, but this time, cancer got the better of him. It had returned to his lungs. Despite our best efforts, he was constantly breathless, so the time had come for palliative care at his new home near Narooma where he had become an oyster farmer, with his partner and her two children. In January 2019, both Michael Boyer and I received a text message from Charles's sister Emma and his brother Jeremy.

Chas is not doing very well & he is clearly not getting any better — his breathing is a huge challenge, made worse by the humidity of summer. He is also incredibly thin. Luckily he is at home living & sleeping in his chair & he is comfortable . . . Of course, Chas is his usually bossy self, keeping everyone in line, so typical!

Charles Hagenbach passed away soon after, on 6 February, having put up a great fight. I think of him every time I see a protea, and they are a favourite bloom of mine to this day.

14

UNDERSTANDING THE ACRONYMS

My passion has always been patients and that's why I remained a clinical nurse practitioner instead of moving into management. Even though every one of my roles had a certain level of management in it, that aspect of the job wasn't really for me – but patients were. I do love research, however, and I think that's how you can change clinical practice. I honestly believe you can make the biggest difference in patient care by asking and observing not only the patient themselves, but how their relatives and friends react. In my time as a cancer nurse I was involved in various studies looking at different combinations of chemotherapy, many of which, as I have indicated before, are highly toxic both to good cells and bad.

In the early days of treating testicular cancer, we used a drug combination known as PVB – platinum (in the form of cisplatin), vinblastine and bleomycin – with a patient having four to six cycles of the regimen every 21 days. The reason why this cancer treatment, or any cancer treatment for that matter, is completed in cycles is to prevent the cancer from growing. We administered platinum on day 1, vinblastine on days 1 and 2, and bleomycin on days 1, 8 and 15, which was shown by the research to maximise the effectiveness of the drugs and reduce side effects. Then the patient had a break before the 21-day cycle started over again, if all was well, that was.

Cisplatin, the platinum element in the regimen, can cause hearing problems, and we needed to conduct a baseline check before starting the drugs. But if a patient complained of tinnitus or hearing loss after taking the drug, we needed to conduct another audiogram. To avoid waiting for those baseline tests, we needed to shortcut the process. To do so, Michael Boyer called neurologist Michael Halmagyi, who organised for an audiologist to show me how to conduct those very simple hearing checks myself. Dr Halmagyi also provided me with a portable machine to use in my cancer unit. (As it happens, I later treated Sue Halmagyi, Dr Halmagyi's wife and the mother of TV chef 'Fast Ed' Halmagyi. Michael could have had Sue treated anywhere but he chose RPA, not because he worked there, but because he genuinely believed it was the facility best suited to getting his wife better. The cancer eventually won, but Ed said that along the way his mother had the privilege of an extraordinary range of medical advice, trial drugs, incredible staff and every comfort and facility you could imagine. Ed later told me, 'We owe a great deal to Lifehouse. It's not simply a place of medicine, it's a place that helps imbue hope.')

Derek Raghavan was blunt about the impact of cisplatin on a patient's hearing. 'Keith,' he said, 'you either send them deaf or cut the platinum and they die.'

The second drug, vinblastine, was administered on days 1 and 2, and often patients would start their treatment on a Friday. But chemotherapy nurses didn't work on Saturdays back then, so on the second day, the vinblastine had to be administered by a registrar. I had quite a few patients call me, concerned about a small ulcer appearing where the IV cannula had been inserted. I was also concerned about IV leakages causing soft tissue damage around the site of the infusion. While not as severe as anthracycline, like Adriamycin, if the vinblastine leaks into the tissue, it can cause major damage, so I wrote one of my first papers on the subject[1], along with other medical professionals and pharmacists, which looked at the tissue damage, known as extravasation, and how to treat it. Based on a study of the highest risk group of patients, it revealed extravasation took a significant amount of treatment to clear up and a long time to heal. So these are the types of patients who need someone to coordinate all their care who knows the treatment well and who is also highly skilled in all these other areas.

We were, however, able to improve this treatment regimen over time. With help from a US study, we found that rather than giving all the cisplatin on day 1, we could split it over five days, which led to a reduction in nausea and vomiting. There was also less audio toxicity so it didn't affect a patient's hearing as much, and the drug was better tolerated by the patient.

In later years, with better research and improved anti-sickness drugs, we were eventually able to treat them as outpatients, allowing them to return home rather than spend days receiving treatment in hospital. Compared to the early days when a diagnosis of testicular cancer almost certainly meant death, today's 96 per cent survival rate is a huge contrast. We also now conduct adjutant therapy in conjunction with primary treat-ment. If a patient does have one testis removed (rarely are both removed) in an operation called orchiectomy, we know there is still a percentage who will later develop metastasis, the spread of cancer cells to new areas of the body, often by way of the lymph system or bloodstream. We now have a Watch Policy where bloods are taken every month, scans every two months, and the patient is followed up for at least 12 months, then for two years after that and so on. This means that if they do relapse after the primary cancer has been removed, we get onto it early and they can start chemotherapy.

Today that three-drug regimen is called PEB: platinum (cisplatin), etoposide and bleomycin, the vinblastine being omitted because of its toxicity and replaced by etoposide, which proved to be superior. The cisplatin and etoposide are adminis-tered on days 1 to 5, the bleomycin on days 1, 8 and 15, and this cycle is repeated every 21 days. Similar to PVB, the patient has four to six cycles of the PEB regimen. But the cyclical nature of the treatment means that while the cancer cells are constantly bombarded, so are other cells, with patients at risk of develop-ing a potentially fatal high fever and very low white cell count known as febrile neutropenia. Today we use a one-off white blood cell stimulant called Pegylated Filgrastim, usually admin-istered on day 6, to help stimulate white cell growth.

Improvement in the composition, administering and safety of chemotherapy drugs is just one of the many changes I have seen, and taken part in, over the years. Another is the move from inpatient care to outpatient care. After its discovery as a potential cancer treatment drug in 1975, the platinum-based compound now known as cisplatin eventually received approval from the

US Food & Drug Administration in 1978. But its introduction proved a turning point in the treatment of testicular cancer, in particular, as well as many other cancers. Although it kills cancer cells, cisplatin also destroys other cells, including red blood cells and platelets, lowers the white blood cell count and can also dramatically alter renal function. In the 1980s and '90s, patients on cisplatin could be in hospital for days on end, hooked up to an IV and pumped with lots of fluid to reduce the risk of renal failure and dehydration. Cisplatin also caused nausea and vomiting in about 90 per cent of cases and that could continue for days after its administration. In effect, while trying to cure patients of a more significant illness, it also made them very, very ill, so it wasn't the best option when it came to patient comfort. While other platinum-based drugs and cisplatin derivatives have since been developed, they have never been able to replace cisplatin, which is still the most effective of all platinum-based drugs – despite its side effects.

'Is there any way I could do this as an outpatient?' I'd be asked as I hooked another patient up to a drip. 'I'm sure one day we can,' I'd often say. After effective anti-sickness medications were developed in the 1980s, they became more common in the 1990s which helped to provide further incentive for those with cancer to be treated as outpatients. A 1998 pilot study at RPA[2] had already demonstrated that cisplatin was safe to use at home. No patient had gone into renal failure and there were only one or two who'd had to come back into hospital. However, a bigger randomised study was required. Meanwhile, my own motivation for more research into how to administer cancer-fighting drugs and anti-sickness medication to outpatients more easily, and with better results, was threefold.

First: it was often difficult to get people into the hospital because of the wait for a bed. I wanted to eliminate that obstacle.

Second: people don't like to be in hospital. They would rather be at home with their loved ones in a comfortable environment if they are being treated.

Third: getting the pathology investigations done on the same day as the treatment was also often difficult and people frequently had to wait for hours for blood counts and liver and kidney function results to come back.

As offering the best in patient care is what I was committed to, treating those with cancer as outpatients was a cause I was fully behind. But first we had to solve multiple problems, including the ones I've already mentioned.

Nausea comes in three stages: anticipatory, acute and delayed. The anticipation comes before treatment has been given, with patients often associating an environment, person or smell with the administration and/or after-effects of the drugs they have experienced before. That experience could mean being in a car or ambulance on the road to the hospital, or the smell of the hospital itself. Nausea could be brought on by seeing a wall that was a similar colour to one at the hospital or being in a particular treatment room. The acute phase is during treatment and up to 24 hours after, while the delayed phase can take place within 24 hours of treatment, or as long as 5–7 days after the drugs have been administered.

I wanted to prove that with the right protocols, chemo drugs and anti-sickness medication could be administered safely to an outpatient, who could then be sent home, so we applied for a grant to fund a randomised crossover trial. And, just as importantly, I wanted to prove that the quality of life of an outpatient would be just as good if not better than that of an inpatient.

Fortunately, we secured $500,000 from the National Health and Medical Research Council (NHMRC), but there was still some apprehension in the medical profession about the trial, with opponents questioning how we'd get all the required fluid into an outpatient if they were going home.

'We don't want people to go into renal failure and then require dialysis,' they said, but the critics gave emerging technology and the outpatients themselves too little credit.

In a 1993 trial of antiemetic or anti-nausea therapy for patients receiving platinum-based chemotherapy[3], we had already been able to show we could control nausea and vomiting by blocking different pathways via different courses of drugs. While that medication deals with the anticipatory and acute phases of cancer therapy, the delayed phase is still a work in progress. One of the other major requirements of being treated at home as an outpatient is how we offer chemotherapy safely, particularly if we are prescribing patients toxic treatments – especially in high doses – then sending them on their way. While cisplatin-based drugs are now used in 40 per cent of cancer treatments, treatment with high doses previously required inpatient admission with overnight hospitalisation.

Fifty-nine patients were eventually chosen for the new study[4], with 53 completing two cycles of high-dose cisplatin (HDC), and while we monitored those patients in hospital, outpatients were encouraged to keep a diary and recollect their side effects so we could help with their recovery at home. We also looked at how many patients bounced back or had to come back into hospital for a longer stay after their outpatient treatment because of other associated medical issues. We looked at the admission rate of people with nausea and vomiting and other health problems, such as fevers and febrile neutropenia (an abnormally low number of neutrophil granulocytes – a type of white blood cell – in the blood). But in the end, there were no significant differences between inpatients and outpatients when it came to rating nausea, vomiting, fatigue, anxiety, depression and overall quality of life. The time given over to professional nursing care was a lot longer for inpatients than it was for outpatients – by almost an hour – and 90 per cent of all patients said they preferred to be an outpatient rather than an inpatient. So the study showed that outpatient treatment was the preferred option, appeared safe and used fewer resources. In addition, patients reported a better quality of life and had fewer overall hospital admissions.

After the success of that study, we were able to negotiate with various hospital departments to have patients receiving chemo-therapy made a second priority – after A&E patients – for both haematology (blood) tests and biochemistry (liver function and kidney function, etc) tests. The turnaround was a lot quicker and although patients would still have to wait at least an hour or more for their results, they could start their fluids in the meantime, meaning we could cut down on the time the patient was at hospital.

With these smoother pathways and depending on the patient, the drugs they required and how they were adminis-tered, we were able to cut out two to three hours of treatment time, per patient. That's a lot of hours. That 2010 randomised crossover trial comparing inpatient and outpatient administra-tion of high-dose cisplatin is now a pivotal study and you'll find it referred to in nearly all cancer institutions throughout the world. It couldn't be clearer in which direction we should go. Quality of life will always win out in my book.

VENOUS ACCESS DEVICES

Venous Access Devices (VADs) are a significant part of the transition from treatment in a hospital to treatment at home. VADs are implantable devices, inserted in the upper chest under the skin and connected to a catheter which leads to a large blood vessel. The VADs allow for the administration of chemo at home, via a special needle, inserted either by a nurse, or, with some training, by the patient themselves. Before the introduction of VADs in the early 1990s, I'd say 90 per cent of people were treated as inpatients while only 10 per cent were treated as outpatients. By the mid-1990s, as beds became more valuable in the health system, it became increasingly hard to get people into hospital for treatment, so part of my role was to look at different chemotherapy regimens to see if there was any way we could give them to people as outpatients.

Along with VADs, the potential for outpatient care at home was dramatically improved by the development of more effective anti-sickness medications, because these would enable us to have more control over the nausea and vomiting that were side effects of the chemo drugs. Those two side effects were a significant hurdle to the treatment of cancer patients at home because if a patient becomes dehydrated as a result of vomiting, then they need to come into Emergency and be connected to IV fluids via a drip. In the worst cases, dehydration can cause renal failure. If we could manage these side effects in a patient's home in addition to giving them their treatment, then we could solve several problems at once.

There were also certain chemo regimens becoming available such as continuous infusion, so if we were able to insert an implantable device, such as a portacath, into a patient, we could then administer the major part of the treatment to them as an outpatient in the clinic, then send the patient home with a pump to continue treatment over several days. A portacath uses a catheter inserted into a vein in the patient's chest via one of two cuts. The catheter or tube is then tunnelled under the skin to the second cut where it is connected to a port which is fitted into a space created under the skin. The drugs are then administered via the port. A written educational package was given to patients and their carers, explaining the care of their pumps and VADs, as well as containing information about their chemotherapy. All patients were required to have a relative or carer who was able to assist them with dressing the catheter line and they also had to understand the mechanics of the infusion pump. Contact numbers for the chemotherapy team, including myself, were given to all patients in case of problems.

In our first study[5], we used a Continuous Ambulatory Delivery Device or CADD-1 pump, which ran on a battery. Unfortunately, the first lot of CADDs we used caused me quite a few headaches. I remember well that first Christmas when they were in use as I was at my sister's house in Miranda, miles away from work, supposedly celebrating with my own family. While the others were opening presents, the only thing I was opening was the urgent messages on my pager. All Christmas Day, patients on chemotherapy in their own homes having drugs administered via these pumps had alarms going off or batteries going dead or they couldn't get a fresh battery into the device. Well, fresh batteries are usually in great demand at that time of year, and while it was not much of a merry Christmas for me, at least the patients got to spend it at home with their loved ones.

I was later introduced to a disposable pump or multiday infuser made by Baxter Healthcare, a local subsidiary of a US company and the manufacturer of intravenous infusion fluids and the devices used to administer them. These continuous pressure pumps consist of a small cylinder with a clear balloon inside. As with the CADD-1 devices, all the individual drug doses were prepared by Baxter, while the RPA pharmacy department was responsible for the coordination and ordering of the CADD-1 cassettes and the Baxter multiday infusers. The infusers don't need a battery, are quite small and a patient can carry one in a bag or on a belt holster. They also work on body temperature, so if a patient's temperature increases, the pumps work faster to administer the drugs in a bid to get the patient's temperature back to normal. Conversely, if a patient's temperature decreases, the pump goes slower. At that stage in their development, the pumps weren't quite as accurate as the battery-operated pumps, but they proved much easier for patients to manage themselves at home. They also enabled a patient to receive treatment at home while having a relatively normal day – within reason – plus using them freed up a hospital bed which otherwise would have been occupied for up to a day or two. While I wouldn't recommend it, one guy even went for a run with his pump attached.

But we also recognised that these were quite toxic drugs being self-administered by novices, so before we tried out this new delivery system we had to test the procedure with patients while they were still inpatients, then write a raft of protocols and procedures before they were able to take home their kit. There was not only a lot of education required of the patients but also their flatmates, relatives and spouses. You needed to train everybody because if something went wrong – and invariably it did – then they would know what to do.

We provided information regarding the safe handling of cytotoxic drugs and instructions for the management of any potential cytotoxic spills. Any equipment necessary for the safe disposal of cytotoxic wastes was also supplied and included a cytotoxic disposal bin for used infusers or CADD pump cassettes. And they didn't go unused. For example, one patient snagged a medication-filled tube on his armchair, tore the tubing from the canister and had his chemotherapy drugs spraying all over his lounge room. Another patient was digging out weeds in his garden – with a pump attached – and got a pitchfork caught around the tube, puncturing it and spraying chemo drugs all around his yard like it was weedkiller. So we had to be strict with patients before sending them home, impressing upon them, 'You've got to look after this.'

We also had to come up with several safety measures, including taping the tubes to an arm and threading the tube through a protective medical sleeve before a patient left the hospital, then we designed these little carry bags for the pumps to keep them safe. In the early days, you could get 24-hour or 48-hour pumps, but later we were able to introduce a pump that infused the drugs over four days. Many cancer patients adapted very quickly, enjoying the freedom that these infusion pumps allowed. Back in the 1990s, I even taught one RPA patient to administer his own drugs and change his portacath needle and pump so he could go on a long holiday to Europe. He owned a villa in the south of France, and because I had connections at the Royal Marsden in London from my time there, the patient would regularly fly over to the UK to get his bloods checked. They'd send the results back to me in Sydney where I would organise for the Marsden to top up his drug treatment, then he'd head back to his villa. We were able to extend his holiday for two months without him having to stop his chemotherapy treatment. But this was no European holiday for me and it's not always that easy to change treatments.

VADs represented a great improvement in our ability to administer cancer treatments, but their use can be associated with risks: specifically, the risk of blood clots. As mentioned, the portacath goes into the upper chest and the catheter is threaded down to the superior vena cava, a big blood vessel and one of the great venous trunks that return deoxygenated blood from the systemic circulation to the right atrium of the heart. A big blood vessel is required to get the drugs through. We conducted quite a few studies in the early days, putting patients on blood thinners such as Warfarin to prevent blood clots, and looking at studies out of the UK, where just one daily milligram of Warfarin would keep the blood a little thinner. Then there was a randomised study looking at no thinning agent or anticoagulant at all versus no treatment or prevention.

Today, on TV, health insurance ads show a nurse going into a home and delivering chemotherapy treatment, with pictures of the patient having fun with their dog or sitting on their porch and they are hooked up to a fairly innocuous-looking device. That's partly because of the work we did 20 to 30 years ago. Back then, we even set up a program called 'Hospital in the Home', but after a couple of years it wasn't cost-effective in the public system because one nurse could only really treat two or three people a day, and then they'd have to go back to see the patient again the following day if they were on multiple-day chemotherapies. Having said that, there are hospitals such as St George and Prince of Wales in Sydney that still have a 'Hospital in the Home' service that delivers chemotherapy to a patient or just administers an injection to a patient at home to save them going into hospital.

★

PERITONEAL DEVICES

The peritoneum is the cavity in which the bowel sits, and people who have different forms of cancer occasionally have a blockage where the peritoneal fluid builds up – as much as 5 to 7 litres – and as a result, there is abdominal swelling. If you are a patient, you may find that a doctor will tap away at your stomach, known as palpating the abdomen, to check if there is fluid, or ascites, build-up. This condition complicates many advanced malignancies and can result in abdominal pain, discomfort, anorexia, nausea and shortness of breath. To relieve the pressure, a procedure called paracentesis is undertaken, where a needle is inserted into the peritoneal space to drain off that fluid and relieve those symptoms in the vast majority of patients. While repeated paracentesis has potential complications, treatment can be time-consuming and requires medical staff, nursing staff and occasionally imaging guidance and/or hospital admission. There were obvious benefits in training nursing staff to conduct the procedure in the outpatients' department and potentially in a patient's home.

However, if the treatment was conducted in a patient's home, it required an implanted, permanent peritoneal port as an alternative to repeated abdominal paracentesis. Our new study[6] suggested that peritoneal port placement was safe, feasible, and resulted in symptomatic improvement for most patients. While further studies comparing safety, convenience, quality-of-life and cost-benefit with standard paracentesis procedures were later required[7], in the palliative care unit peritoneal ports were the preferred option for the symptomatic treatment of malignant ascites. Peritoneal devices are now used across the spectrum, including for the administration of chemotherapy into the peritoneum for ovarian cancer.

15

FRIENDS, FAMILY AND FOOD FOR THOUGHT

Alongside my nursing and research, I have met many people who have made a big impact on my life. In 1952, 20-year-old Dante Ferzoco stepped off a ship carrying migrants from Italy and headed straight to North Queensland to cut cane for two years before returning to NSW. There he worked as a cook on the Snowy Mountains Scheme, using skills he had picked up while in Rome after the war. Dante had saved enough money to bring his childhood sweetheart, Anna, to Australia, and she arrived four years after he did, having married him by proxy while she was still in Corfinio, their village a few hundred kilometres east of Rome. When I moved to Drummoyne, a suburb in the inner west of Sydney, in 1991, Anna and Dante were there to greet me and have been there for me ever since. Our meeting happened like this.

'I think I might have someone interested in your Balmain place,' my friend Michele told me after I had made mention that I wanted something bigger than my little worker's cottage in Lawson Street, Balmain. As much as I loved my first home, which I bought in 1983, two years after my return from London, it was very small and the street was narrow, and there was no off-street parking. It was time to move. Michele came through with a buyer, a community nurse, who came to see the Balmain cottage straight away.

'I love it! I'll buy it,' she said, and we agreed on a price there and then. But I needed a long settlement, because at that point, I hadn't been able to find anything else to buy. I looked at 68 properties before I bought in Drummoyne.

At first glance, the house had no appeal whatsoever. The bathroom had shag carpet on the floor, an old green enamel bath and awful tiles on the walls. The kitchen was tiny. But the bedrooms and living room were generous, with 14-foot ceilings, and they still had many of the original period features. The house needed a lot of work – a proper bathroom and new kitchen for starters, as well as new guttering and downpipes, a new driveway and repairs to a collapsed fence out the front which was falling down. The sellers kept lowering the price, so after a while, the agent rang me.

'If you are really interested they could do a deal,' she said, but I wasn't convinced. So she spoke to the owners again. They'd already bought a property in Carlingford so needed to sell urgently, and I needed to buy as I had already sold in Balmain. The property stars aligned. The owners brought the price down to a sum I was happy with, and I've never looked back. While the house was a real work in progress for a long time, it was in a fantastic street and close to a church and shops. And even though I had a bridge to cross to get to work,

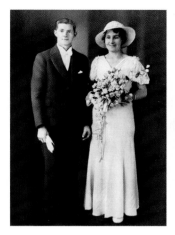

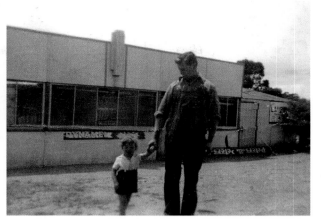

My parents Bill and Pansy Cox on their wedding day in 1934.

Here I am with Dad outside our Cullerin shop, in the early 1950s, prior to the petrol bowsers. I must have been about three in this picture.

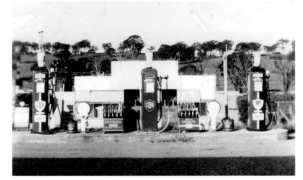

Cullerin General Store showing the new bowsers, probably in the 1950s. We were the only service station between Gunning and Goulburn. Cars would line up to get a refill.

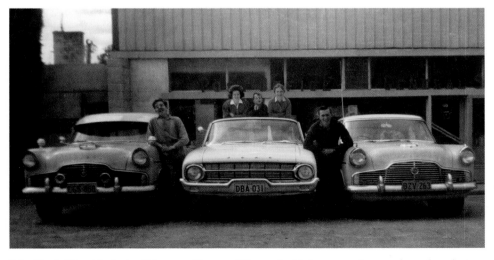

Me (far left) with Judy, Vincent, Ret and Ronnie. Brian must have taken the photo. Both Brian and Ronnie had Zephyrs and Dad's Ford Falcon utility is in the middle.

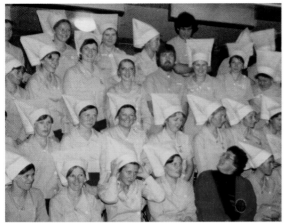

Me graduating as Keith 'Dorsett' Cox with my class, which includes flatmates Belinda Chapman on my left and Barb Maitland on my right. The only other male nurse, Kim Skinner, is behind me.

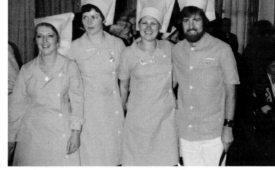

Me in a borrowed veil that the female nurses used to wear, with (from left) Barb, Leslie Earl and Belinda.

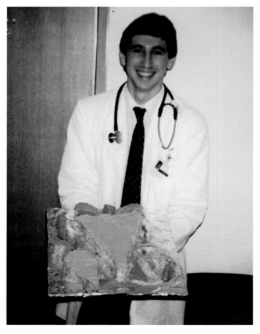

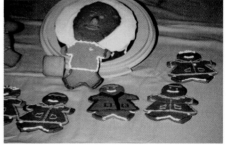

Above: Keith and the Chemettes in gingerbread form, made by Tim Driscoll, now Professor of Epidemiology and Occupational Medicine at Sydney University.

Left: A very youthful Michael Boyer presents carrot cake at the weekly competition. Michael now heads up Chris O'Brien Lifehouse at RPA.

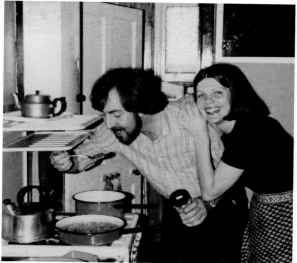

We entertained many friends in our London flat throughout 1980–81, including my favourite Royal Marsden classmate, Sarah.

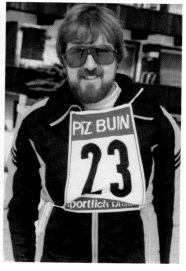

I competed at Kitzbühel in 1980, on one of my many ski trips, but broke the finish pole – with my nose.

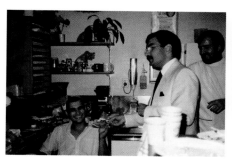

At one of our annual RPA Christmas parties in the 1980s, Derek Raghavan presented Charles Hagenback with Patient of the Year award.

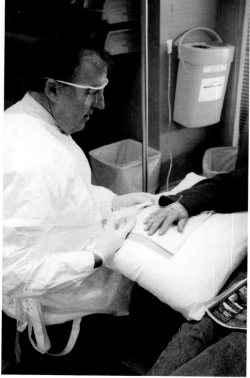

Administering chemotherapy in the 1990s. While I did wear gloves, goggles and a Tyvek gown, notice the absence of a mask.

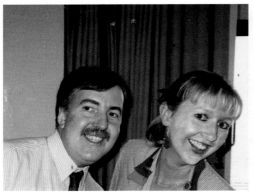

With my E9 Special Unit second–in–command Tish in the 1990s.

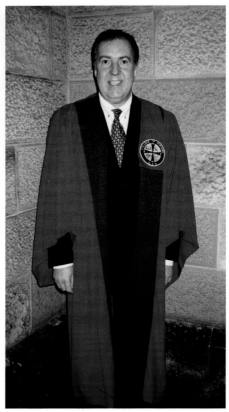

I was inducted as a member of the NSW College of Nursing at the Great Hall, Sydney University, in the mid–1990s after two decades of nursing.

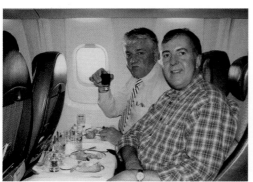

Dining onboard the Concorde with Christofle cutlery, a set of which one of my charges took home to Nowra.

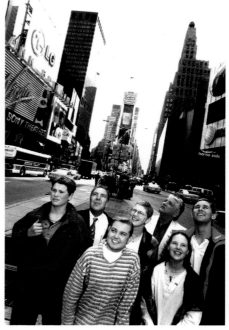

In Times Square with the CanTeen crew.

© Alex Towle

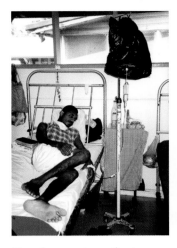

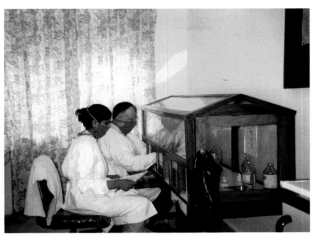

Treating mute patient Simon on my trip to PNG.

The old-fashioned hood at BP Koirala Memorial Hospital in Chitwan, Nepal. We later jerry-rigged an exhaust extraction system.

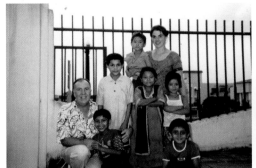

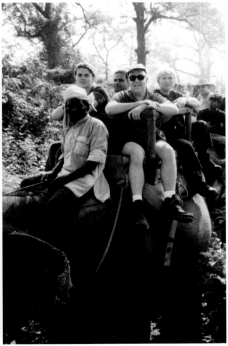

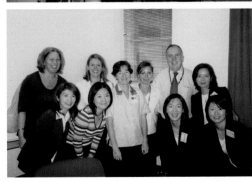

Top left: The children who came to greet Kate and me every afternoon in Nepal. We had their clothes washed and bathed them just before we left.

Right: On an elephant ride in the Chitwan National Park during some leisure time in Nepal.

Bottom left: With students from a course for Japanese cancer nurses which ran for several years at the Sydney Cancer Centre during the early 2000s.

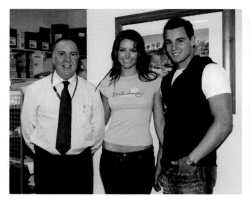

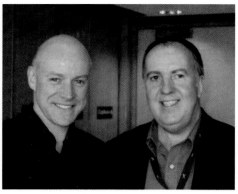

With then-reigning Miss Universe, Jennifer Hawkins, and her partner, Jake Wall, while touring the Sydney Cancer Centre in 2004 after she made a susbtantial financial donation.

Opera singer Anthony Warlow and I after he closed the International Cancer Nursing Conference in Sydney in 2004.

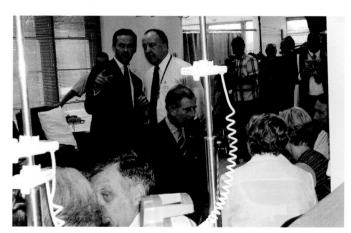

He wants to talk to those guys up the end! Talking with a royal minder while His Royal Highness Prince Charles visits the Sydney Cancer Centre in 2005.

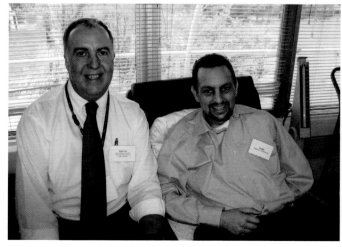

With Doug Yorath during the Royal visit.

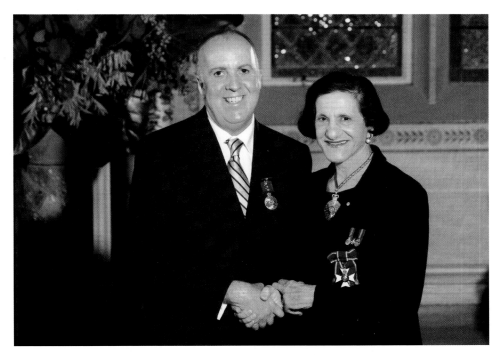

With NSW Governor Marie Bashir after I received my OAM.

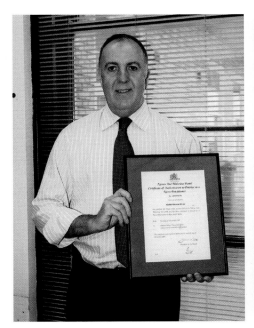

With my nurse practitioner certificate in 2006. I was only the third cancer nurse practitioner in Australia, but the first male.

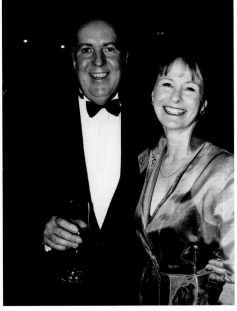

With Gail O'Brien at a Sydney Cancer Centre fundraiser for Lifehouse, after the death of her husband Chris O'Brien.

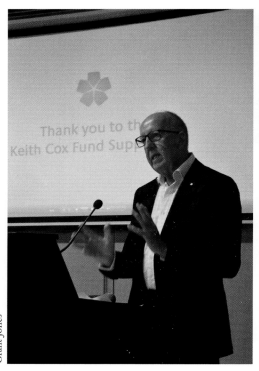

Grant Jones

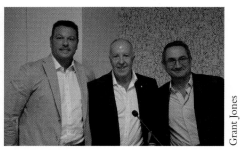

Grant Jones

Above: Cancer survivors and financial contributors Julian Hofer and David Boyer were my guests at the launch of the Keith Cox OAM Clinical Education Fund on International Nurses Day in 2019.

Left: At the 2019 launch of the Keith Cox OAM Clinical Education Fund, 18 months after Gail called me in Italy to ask if I'd accept a scholarship named after me.

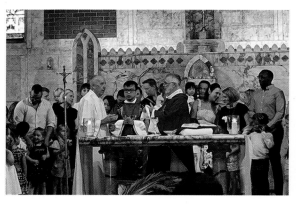

Serving as an acolyte at
St Mark's Church,
Drummoyne.

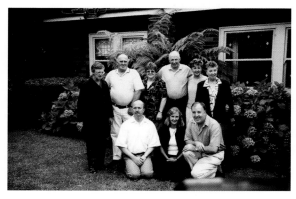

The Cox siblings (standing, left to right) Dawn, Ronald, Judith, Brian, Coral, Fay (Sister Chrys), and (bottom row, from left), Vincent, Loretta and myself. Taken in the 1990s at Vincent's Blue Mountains home.

it wasn't that far from Royal Prince Alfred in the scheme of things.

I don't know if you've ever bought and sold a house on the same day, but it often has a domino effect, with your property settlement relying on the sale or otherwise of another property. All told, on Friday, 8 March 1991, there were eight other settlements somehow connected to the sale of my little Balmain cottage. While the Balmain house was being settled, I only had access to my new house keys after 2 pm. So I gathered a few of my hospital friends – Ann Mills, a secretary, and her builder husband and Michele – who said they'd help me clean my new, much bigger Federation home in Drummoyne before I moved in. We arrived at the house armed with mops, buckets and cleaning chemicals, and started to wash the walls with sugar soap and clean the floors to make everything ready for furniture to be moved in the following day. We were hard at work when Dante, accompanied by Anna, poked his head through the open door. 'Hello, we're Dante and Anna and we live next door. Welcome,' he said cheerily. We have been good neighbours ever since.

After all our cleaning, Michele and I and the rest of the cleaning crew celebrated with fish and chips from Ocean Foods, eating and drinking wine while sitting on the now clean dining room floor. That night, completely exhausted, I went back to Balmain and packed up my old home. The next day the removalists came and we got the move done pretty quickly, but even after we moved all my stuff into Drummoyne, the new place still looked very, very empty.

The year I moved in next door to Dante and Anna, it was just the two of them in their big two-storey house. About

18 months before, their youngest daughter Lety had married Frank and the young couple had moved into their own place. Lety's older sister Maurizia was already living in Mauritius after marrying a veterinary surgeon there, while Dante and Anna's only son, also called Frank, was living out west. Because there was just the pair of them in this big house that had once been filled with kids, they now sought company and we got to know each other well.

In those days there was a well-tended veggie garden in Dante and Anna's backyard and they often had family and friends over. Dante was always cooking. I'd come home late after some very long hours and I would often have skipped lunch or only grabbed a sandwich at my desk while trying to catch up on emails. I'd be pulling into my driveway at night and there they would be at their own front door: 'Keith! We've got dinner here for you.' By the time I put my key in the door, they would be there at my doorstep with a warm meal. Back then, Dante worked at Balmain Hospital as a cook, and his meals were delicious, while Anna worked at Tuta, a hospital supplies manufacturer in Lane Cove. Dante would start early and finish about 2 pm, and when he arrived home, he'd always cook dinner for Anna and make extra for me.

I consider Anna and Dante to be my second parents, and Anna would often introduce me to people as her adopted son. Having lost my father when I was 32, I had missed a listening ear, fatherly advice and the care and compassion that a parent offers. I have also been there for Dante more often of late as we lost Anna to cancer in 2017 and Dante is getting older and needs my help. I will be there for him, too, when it's time to say our final goodbye.

JULIAN HOFER'S ONGOING DONATIONS
(SURVIVOR)

Professor Jim Bishop had been appointed the first director of the Sydney Cancer Centre when it was established in 1996. Jim came from Peter MacCallum Cancer Centre in Melbourne, where he was head of cancer services. Based in E9 North Block of RPA, the centre was founded on best practice principles in cancer treatment and incorporated the cancer services of RPA and Concord Repatriation hospitals and the inpatient palliative care unit at Canterbury Hospital. As demand for specialist cancer services grew, the centre expanded to accommodate several floors in Gloucester House, a six-storey brick building originally constructed in 1936 which featured an art deco–style front door and terrazzo flooring. It was conveniently located next door to RPA and we would eventually take over the whole building.

It was 1996, the same year the Sydney Cancer Centre was established, when Julian Hofer became a patient at Gloucester House just before he turned 24. He had been diagnosed with Stage 4 Hodgkin's lymphoma and was referred to oncologist Michael Boyer by Dr Andrew Korda, the father of a friend of Julian's. The introduction was not by Julian's choice but was one that, in hindsight, he would be eternally grateful for. Michael Boyer was just 36 at the time, and when they met Julian felt an immediate connection to, confidence in and empathy from Michael. Julian knew he was in the right hands.

In the Sydney Cancer Centre, Julian was scheduled for fortnightly chemotherapy treatment over six months, with a drug regimen of Adriamycin, bleomycin, vinblastine and dacarbazine – a pretty strong combination otherwise known as ABVD.

Before his treatment, Julian had to undergo several other clinical tests and it was during this process that I was introduced to him. He would later come to call me his 'cancer concierge'. Julian soon discovered that as a cancer patient there is a huge amount of stress, anxiety and vulnerability that comes with treatment. As a nurse, I was able to help recognise his emotional needs, calm his fears and also help him come to terms with the cancer journey that lay ahead. Julian once asked out loud, 'Why me?' and we often spoke about it. My response was: 'Why not you? Cancer doesn't discriminate.'

I made sure I was there during his appointments and was always available for a chat and a cup of tea before or after his treatment. I'd mark his blood tests as urgent, prior to chemotherapy, so he wouldn't have to spend too much of his day in the hospital. I knew all the tricks, too, and while he may not have been thinking about it then, I called him to say he needed to make a 'donation at the bank'. As Julian recalled in his speech at my retirement function:

> *Keith escorted me up to the old maternity building, as he did with many of my appointments, up to the fertility clinic area where I was handed a small sample jar and a brown paper bag. Keith pointed me towards a room across the hallway and gave me the following instructions: 'Now Jules: when you get inside, make sure you press the "Occupied" light on the wall so that no one interrupts you. In the top drawer, there are a couple of naughty magazines, and on the back of the door, there is a full-size poster of a beautiful naked woman with long hair.'*
>
> *I entered the room and was greeted by the smell of hospital strength Domestos, and my first sight was an old chair that had*

been re-covered in thick, clear plastic, a small TV that wouldn't turn on, and some very late '70s-esque brown carpentry. I pressed the 'do not disturb' button, as instructed, and shut the door, and there she was! The beautiful naked woman Keith spoke of, in all her glory, with her long hair ... that hair ... absolutely EVERYWHERE.

I then headed over to the drawers to find two crinkled old magazines (clearly well-read) circa 1977, filled with women with similar hairstyles! It was clear that the current material was going to have very little benefit to the task at hand! I emerged six weeks later ...

By some miracle (another Keith miracle perhaps?) my donation was a success! I headed to the counter to make my 'deposit', and was greeted by a lady wearing a full-length white gown, complete with mask, and robotic hand claw that enabled her to stand three metres away from me to collect my sample. I quickly departed, hoping no one had seen me, but that big red light outside the 'donation room' was a big giveaway. Turns out while the donation was a success, for some reason that sample wasn't adequate and I had to repeat the process, somewhat ironic.

The second procedure Julian needed to have done ahead of chemotherapy was a bone-marrow biopsy. While it is a rather unpleasant procedure to endure, this particular investigation was due to take place on Julian's 24th birthday. Julian has the build of a rugby player and I stood next to him, holding his hand as he lay on the gurney. I gave the attending doctor strict instructions.

'It's Jules's birthday, and he is NOT to feel any pain. Give him 10 milligrams of midaz.'

Now midazolam is a very short-acting drug, similar to Valium or lorazepam, but rather than being given orally it is given intravenously so it works quickly. When the drug took effect, Julian started laughing and chatting, oblivious of what was to occur. A registrar then braced himself against an awake and fully conscious, but partially delirious, Julian. With his knee on Julian's bed, the registrar was trying with his full force to extract the bone marrow sample required. Meanwhile, I was on the opposite side of the bed trying to keep Julian – and the registrar – from falling off. While the drilling in of a very large needle and the sucking out of the bone marrow is very, very painful, Julian later said he didn't feel a thing. I think I was probably more traumatised than he was.

Over the next seven months of chemo and radiation, and the following ten-plus years of follow-up checks, Julian and I developed a friendship that goes far beyond a patient–nurse relationship. After his recovery, he went on to become a very successful trader in the financial markets and lived in Dubai for a time, making his money in the international gold market. So when I was on an overnight stopover in Dubai on my way to a conference in Europe, Julian got in touch with his contacts there and organised for me to be picked up at the airport, taken to a fancy hotel and then had the car return the following day and take me back to the airport. Julian has since made several donations – the financial type – to the Keith Cox Scholarship, which Chris O'Brien's widow Gail helped set up, an education fund that goes towards learning and development for nursing and allied health staff at Chris O'Brien Lifehouse. Our friendship continues to this day, as Julian recalled in his speech at my retirement:

He is my friend. As hard as my cancer journey was, I learnt so much about myself, but more than that, Keith taught me about true compassion, kindness, and empathy. I would not change this period of my life. Keith was never far from my side during my treatment.

FRED HOLLOWS (1929–1993)

Famous eye surgeon Fred Hollows had been diagnosed with renal cancer in the late '80s and already had a kidney removed, but his prognosis had looked pretty good. After being diagnosed, he said: 'Why should I be spared cancer when so many other people have it?'

But by the early 1990s, Fred had relapsed and his cancer metastasised, so he came to see us at RPA. Derek Raghavan was then the urogenital oncologist at RPA and asked me to get involved in his care. Fred came in every three weeks or so for chemotherapy and radiotherapy, so I saw him fairly regularly and got to know both him and his delightful wife, Gabi, very well. While we didn't encourage children in the ward, the couple had twin girls, toddlers still in a stroller at the time, so I was able to meet them too when Gabi dropped Fred off for treatment.

Fred was already very well known by then, and I could tell he really wanted to make a difference in the world, which is another reason why we got on so well. We had the same passion to help people, and while his passion was eye surgery and his legacy lives on, mine is cancer care and, hopefully, my legacy will live on too. When we first met, I had to go through his chemotherapy treatment with him to tell him what was involved and what side effects there were. When we talked about general things, he always had a good sense of humour, and never once complained about his predicament. He was one of the loveliest patients – and people – I have ever come into contact with. In the end, he was accepting of his own impending death, saying: 'I don't think dying's such a terrible business ... I've had a fair suck of the pomegranate.'

During those visits, he was always very chatty and told me about his projects around the world. He had been on TV often to talk about the work he was doing in Nepal, conducting cataract surgery on everyone from children to the elderly through a very simple operation that enabled them to see again. He had already raised millions in funding and also persuaded other Australian doctors to become involved by training local eye doctors in Nepal. According to Fred, what he saw as a simple operation made a massive difference to the lives of those who were fortunate enough to undergo it. While I was still learning and gaining knowledge about cancer care, I saw Fred as an inspiration to learn more and do more for less fortunate people.

While Fred eventually set in motion the training of local surgeons, he sadly never got to see the Eritrean and Nepalese lens factories that have gone on to produce millions of cost-effective intraocular lenses for cataract surgeries in more than 70 countries.

Professor Fred Hollows died at his home in Randwick, aged 63, on 10 February 1993.

Learning of Fred's 'eye-opening' work from the man himself would later lead me to my own Nepalese adventure.

★

I've been lucky to meet so many wonderful people and make lifelong friends in and outside of the hospital. Time goes quickly when you spend it with people who matter to you, whether they are family or friends.

In the winter of 1999, there were two big events to celebrate my 50th birthday. My sister Ret and my brother-in-law, Tony, held a sit-down dinner for 50 guests in Miranda on a Saturday night. We had drinks around their pool which had been dotted with bamboo lanterns so it looked like a tropical lagoon, then we feasted in their garage, which they had disguised with raw calico draped over the walls and ceiling. It was a glorious night. The following day, my RPA oncology colleague and friend Annabelle Child and her husband John held a lunch for me at their house in Lane Cove. They'd rearranged their dining and sitting room to seat 38 friends and colleagues. It was at that lunch that my good friend Tish played taped messages from colleagues around the world and read from a booklet, *Keith Cox: This Is Your Life*, which she had compiled and printed. Tish read out many passages from the book, which made me blush with embarrassment, including Derek Raghavan's recall of my expertise in cannulation.

My earliest recollections of this old fellow (Keith) are his associations with MAGIC. When I was an intern (1974) covering Blackburn Pavilion at night, Keith was a senior enrolled nurse. I was untalented in my first weeks (and subsequently) at finding veins in patients who were having seizures, and after the requisite multiple efforts, would go and seek support from Mr Cox. I would describe the misery that the patient and I were sharing, and Keith would suggest that I have one more go, and if I felt it was not a great

139

success, to leave the IV cannula in place, let him know, and go and take a short break. I would do so, and ALWAYS, when I returned, the cannula would be just where I had left it (more or less), but in a vein and with an IV running: MAGIC!!!

It was a wonderful celebration and the nickname 'King of Cannulation' would stick with me for many years.

16

LOSING PATIENCE IN PNG

By 2030, the World Health Organization (WHO) expects that 70 per cent of all cancer deaths will be in developing countries. WHO also lists Papua New Guinea as having the highest rate of cancer in the Pacific region, recording 11,000 cancer cases per year and 7500 cancer deaths a year – that's more than 20 per day! Back in June 2000, I went to PNG with radiation therapist Chris Carney as part of an AusAID-sponsored trip to help train nurses there in cancer care. To say it was an eye-opener, in a country just a short flight away from Australia, is an understatement.

We landed in Port Moresby and were met by a local representative of AusAID, as it was then known, which was part of the Australian Government's Department of Foreign Affairs and Trade. An Australian AusAID representative took us to our hotel complex, which was in a compound surrounded by barbed-wire fences and guarded by a security officer who patrolled the perimeter with an Alsatian dog. It was a bit confronting.

141

The day after we arrived, I went to Port Moresby Hospital to look at the cancer services there and evaluate the facilities – or lack thereof – and write a report for AusAID. We were in Port Moresby for just three days, so I wanted to do as much as I could while I was there, meeting doctors, nurses and other medical staff before I was due to head off to the National Cancer Centre at Angau Hospital in Lae. There I was to teach classes on cancer care and to meet and treat patients. First off, at Port Moresby Hospital, I was introduced to a local oncologist who was in charge of cancer services at the hospital, and I was then taken on a brisk tour of the inpatient ward before I headed off to the outpatients. It was here I met a young nurse. We started to talk about her training and which department she had come from, and she admitted she had come from operating theatres.

'The nurse that was here left so they asked me to do chemotherapy,' she told me, adding that she had no idea about working in oncology or using chemotherapy drugs, and really no clue how to treat cancer patients at all. She then cut the conversation short, saying she needed to administer chemotherapy to a patient.

'So, have you had much training in the administration of chemotherapy?' I asked her before we headed off to collect the prepared drugs. 'None,' said the theatre nurse. I asked her where she mixed them. 'Just here,' she said, pointing to a room. The particular cocktail she was preparing is called CMF, which she was using in the treatment of breast cancer. The C stands for cyclophosphamide and M for methotrexate, while F stands for fluorouracil. I said: 'Do you give the methotrexate as a bolus injection and the cyclophosphamide as an infusion?'

She looked at me oddly. 'Oh, no!' she said. 'I just mix it all in the one bag or the one bottle.'

'All in the one bottle?' I asked, astonished. A bolus injection should usually be given in a single, large dose when a patient needs something like methotrexate or fluorouracil circulating through the bloodstream almost immediately, while in those days cyclophosphamide, also called Cytoxan, was usually given orally over 14 days or as an IV.

I was shocked at first that they used the old-fashioned glass IV bottles, not the plastic Solupak bags as we had been using for decades. These drugs are all very toxic in their own right, but who knows what happens when you put them all together in the one bottle? The drugs in this cocktail could easily have had a chemical reaction with each other in the wrong conditions. It was not the way I was used to seeing it done. It made me realise that while Papua New Guinea is not very far from Australia, just 5 kilometres or a 15-minute boat ride separating Saibai Island in Australia from the PNG mainland, a span of almost 30 years divides us when it comes to the standard of medical treatment. I just couldn't get my head around it.

The trip to Port Moresby was over quickly, then we flew straight to Lae. If I'd thought Port Moresby was primitive, Lae was something else entirely. Up in the Highlands, and an hour's flight away, Lae has the much bigger National Cancer Centre, which then included an old, second-hand cobalt-60-therapy machine that didn't work. Now, a cobalt-60-therapy machine is commonly used for external beam radiation treatments for patients with cancer and delivers high-energy gamma rays to a patient's tumour. These treatments are designed in such a way that they destroy the cancer cells while sparing the surrounding normal tissue. It seemed odd that Lae, over 300 kilometres from the capital across mountainous terrain, had the only cobalt-60-therapy machine in the whole of PNG. It remains the only one in the country, albeit one that still does not work.

We arrived on a Thursday but I wasn't starting the cancer nursing courses until Monday, so the staff suggested we tour the hospital and the cancer ward in particular. This hospital had a whole ward of cancer patients, probably about 25. As expected, conditions were fairly primitive, at least by Australian standards, and the staff had very little idea or training in oncology or cancer care or, moreover, my specialty of chemo-therapy treatment. The hospital in Lae took me back to the Florence Nightingale wards of old with bed after bed down a long corridor. The beds were aluminium and the drip stands were covered in chipped white enamel, all in front of walls that had probably last been painted decades ago. The floors were concrete and ventilation was via ancient ceiling fans. A couple of my uncles had fought in PNG in World War II and I imagined it looked something like what they might have seen. I was also quite shocked to see staff sitting in the nurses' room at one end of a ward, tearing off little bits from a big wad of cotton wool to make their own cotton wool balls. After a brief tour, we were introduced to the patients includ-ing one young chap by the name of Simon, who was just 24.

'Keith, can you do anything for this young fellow?' I was asked. Simon had already been subjected to a laryngectomy, or having his voice box removed, so he couldn't speak. After the laryngectomy, he had been taken to Lae from his home in Port Moresby to have radiotherapy via the only radiother-apy machine in the country. Most head and neck cancers don't spread outside the head and neck region, but as his cancer was spreading locally to some nodes in his neck, it was hoped the radiotherapy treatment would halt that. But the day after Simon arrived in Lae, the old cobalt-60 machine had broken down – yet again – so there was no radiotherapy to be had. Simon was emaciated and had been at the hospital for weeks without treatment. I found him lying on top of an old bed being fed by a tube in his nose. He looked like the nicest fellow, and even though he couldn't speak to me I asked him, 'Would you like me to help? To give you some chemotherapy?' His eyes lit up and his lips moved; you could see that he was pleading with me. Then he put his thin hand out and grabbed mine and squeezed it. I knew I had to try to help him.

The drug treatment we would have used back at RPA would have been a combination of cisplatin and fluorouracil, with the fluorouracil given as a continuous infusion over four days.

'Do you have these drugs here?' I asked a doctor, and was taken to the outpatient area to be shown a grey metal cabinet. The drugs inside had long expired. So I went around to the pharmacy and was surprised to meet an Englishwoman, highly trained and a very experienced pharmacist.

'What would happen if I gave Simon these expired drugs?' I asked, brandishing the vials.

'How old are they?' she asked. The cisplatin had expired four months ago and the fluorouracil three months ago.

'They may not work because the efficacy of the drug is not as good, but they won't do somebody any harm,' she said, so we decided to give it a try. But I also needed anti-sickness medication to combat the nauseating effects of the cisplatin. Because Simon was already so thin, we needed to make sure we controlled any vomiting. As he'd had a laryngectomy, vomiting would also have been quite difficult for him. The best thing they could come up with was metoclopramide or Maxolon, a dopamine antagonist or antiemetic, and they also had dexamethasone which we knew, in combination with other anti-sickness medication, helps delay nausea and vomiting in the administration of platinum-based drugs such as cisplatin.

I went back to Simon and explained everything to him, and while I presume he did not understand all of it, he seemed to get a rough idea. Using his eyes and lips to communicate, Simon demonstrated that he would like to give it a go. His permission was one of the things I needed before I was prepared to give the treatment. But I thought to myself, just imagine the headlines back home – 'AUSSIE CANCER NURSE KILLS PATIENT IN PNG' – because I was giving this guy expired drugs and didn't have good anti-sickness medication. But what choice did he or I have? So I told the doctor that I wanted a full blood count and biochemistry profile, to look at Simon's kidney function test, his white cells, red cells and platelets to see how his liver was. We took the bloods and sent them off to pathology. I was planning to check the results and start treatment the following day.

In between all of this, I was trying to run a five-day course of cancer lectures. It was not only a course for nurses – there were doctors and allied health people in the class as well, 76 in all. I was lecturing from eight thirty in the morning until four o'clock in the afternoon, plus juggling Simon's cancer treatment, then seeing other patients after that, then heading back to another razor-wired hotel compound. And every night I'd be up studying the textbooks until 11 or 12 o'clock, making sure

I knew everything I could on the focus subject before lecturing about it the following day.

There were also some unexpected teething problems. On the first day of lectures, while most of the attendees were very attentive, after lunch they were very slow in returning to the lecture room. I discovered that they were out chewing betelnut or 'buai'. The nut is chewed with a stick of mustard and slaked lime powder or calcium hydroxide which is derived from crushed coral. It is a common stimulant in PNG, and while chewing betelnut is highly addictive, it is also known to cause mouth cancers. I suppose it was the equivalent of the old RPA days when doctors walked into wards with lit pipes, and RPA nurses – including myself – ducked out to smoke in the courtyard. But I was still frustrated that half the class would come back an hour or so late.

'What will I do?' I asked one of the nurse educators.

'Keith, it's PNG time. You'll have a nervous breakdown if you keep worrying about it.'

So, I rewrote the program there and then, developing some mini-workshops for the afternoon sessions and training up some local people to deliver them. Not only did I want them to take ownership, but it would also help spread the load and they would be able to better communicate the information on the overhead slides I was using.

The next day, about 24 hours after Simon's blood was taken, I went down to the ward and asked what his count was like. I was told the bloods weren't back yet and they would probably come through 'any minute'. But no blood count had come through by the end of that day, so the next morning, before I started my lecture, I went down to the ward to check again. 'They're not back yet,' I was told, and this time I decided this was just not good enough. We were into day three, I was leaving the following Monday, and if we were to treat this fellow, I needed the blood results. I was not prepared to treat Simon without them.

While Chris, the radiation therapist, had been to New Guinea before and had given me an idea of what to expect, the attitude and the conditions still shocked me. I also had to explain to Simon that I needed to have the blood results before we started treating him – and I was visiting him twice a day. While Simon had expressive eyes, he couldn't speak to me, so I couldn't tell if he was getting more anxious about the possibility of not being treated. I explained to him about the delay in the blood results and decided to go down to Pathology to check for myself as I wanted to see what the hold-up was. This time I asked one of the local doctors to accompany me to see if they could better communicate the urgency of the issue.

'I sent the blood down on Monday, I was hoping to start treatment on Tuesday and now it's Wednesday and we still don't have the blood results,' I said to the person in Pathology. I was told that the technician who delivered the test results wasn't there. Well, I had seen this type of testing machine before, so I walked over and said: 'Give me the bloods because I know how to do it. You put them on this end of the machine, press the button and it sucks it up, then analyses the blood, and you get the results at this end.'

'Oh no, no, you can't do that! He'll be back any minute!' I was assured. So I said, 'I'm waiting here until he returns,' and I grabbed a chair, sat down, crossed my arms and waited. About two minutes later a young fellow came in, so I said, 'Can you run these bloods for me?' 'Yeah,' he said. 'So, what's the hold-up?' I asked, and he said: 'Oh, I don't know.' It was a mystery.

Before I left Pathology, I watched over him as he put Simon's bloods in the machine, then I headed back at afternoon tea time to find the results waiting for me. It was very frustrating, but it was just the way things were done there.

It was too late to start the treatment that day because you need to give a patient pre-hydration and post-hydration on this regimen. But I was able to tell Simon that based on his blood results I was happy to proceed with his treatment in the morning. So I went back to the ward first thing the next day and asked a doctor to put a cannula in, and we started Simon's pre-hydration. Then I went back during my morning break to check if he was passing urine and was well hydrated, which he was, so I hung the cisplatin in a bag to administer it myself. Now, cisplatin is light sensitive, so it has to be covered and protected from harsh light, but the only thing I could find to put over the top of it was a black garbage bag. *So be it*, I thought. Simon started his cisplatin treatment and we also gave him some high-dose Maxolon and some dexamethasone as his anti-sickness medication. I went back at lunchtime to make sure his urine output was OK and that he wasn't too nauseated. He'd finished the cisplatin and was on his post-hydration, along with the fluorouracil as a continuous infusion. I felt very satisfied with the day's work, but I knew this was just one person in a whole country with a deadly cancer rate.

The doctors were happy that something was being done for Simon and when they saw the positive results from his treatment, they came up to me and said: 'Oh, Keith, now can you come and see this 22-year-old woman who has just come down from the Highlands with Stage 4 cervical cancer?' So I went to see this poor girl, sent down to Lae so she could be given some palliative radiotherapy only to find the machine was broken. Her case looked hopeless; she was likely to die within the next few days or weeks, at best. She didn't speak any pidgin English, so I had to tell the medical staff who were with her that we couldn't do anything but offer her pain relief and make the last couple of days of her journey as comfortable as possible. It would have been devastating for her to come all that way in an obviously painful and advanced condition only to find that we couldn't offer her much of anything. There was talk of sending some of these patients to Townsville for radiotherapy, but even with dozens of available flights or the millions of dollars in healthcare given to PNG, it was a very rare occurrence. I was to discover that the money was not going to the patients who needed it; much of it disappeared (and still does) before it reached them. Supplied drugs sat on the wharf because the government wouldn't pay to move them, and there was no one to service the cancer therapy machines.

As I neared the end of my stay and Simon was finishing his treatment, I used to go and see him four or five times a day. There were a few tears when we said goodbye and I gave him a cap that I had brought with me. As he could read English, I also gave him a novel that I hadn't had time to start. I gave nearly all my clothes to the gardeners at the hospital, and I left all my lecture material with the hospital, so I came home with not much at all except a very sad impression of the care that Papua New Guineans were likely to be offered should they be unlucky enough to get cancer. I doubt either Simon or the young woman with cervical cancer would have survived; they likely died soon after my visit. I had to submit a report when I came back. AusAID sent me a letter of thanks and that was it.

A couple of years later, Professor Martin Tattersall, head oncologist at RPA, and another doctor, Alan Langlands, a radiation oncologist at Westmead Hospital, went to PNG and conducted a similar review, but more on the medical side of cancer treatment than the nursing side. Martin told me that things hadn't improved very much at all. The medical staff were a little bit more knowledgeable, hopefully, after my lectures, both about the policies and guidelines I offered to staff as well as the proper handling of cytotoxic drugs. Despite many promises from the PNG government, according to an October 2019 report, the Lae radiation machine was still out of action and has been since 2016.

But the trip to PNG was a real turning point for me because I thought, *Here am I, lucky to be born in Australia, to have a roof over my head, to be educated. I have so much and these people have so little.* So the next year, in 2001, a period of dramatic change across the globe, I flew to Nepal to undertake similar work.

17

THE MANY SMILING
FACES OF NEPAL

To me, sharing the skills I have learned over the decades has been an important part of giving back as a nurse and cancer nurse practitioner. Whether it is taking to the lectern to offer my views at a cancer conference in Vienna or New York, or visiting patients and educating nurses in a remote hospital in a developing country, it gives me a great deal of fulfilment knowing that I have passed on what I have learned. It was an example set by my mentor, the late Professor Martin Tattersall. Alongside the many other achievements of his career, he travelled the world, including to war-torn Iraq, helping where he could, to educate medical staff in cancer treatment. So, when Pat Cho, an RPA registrar who later became an oncologist, emailed me to ask if I'd head to another far-flung destination, it was hard to say no.

Keith, you wouldn't be interested in coming up and doing some stuff in Nepal, would you? Because all the stuff they want me to do is chemotherapy and how to give it, it's all your type of thing, she wrote. Of course, I replied: *Yes, I'd love to.*

I made plans, took time off and was due to fly out on 13 September 2001, but two days before that, the world changed. While almost everything was put on hold because of 9/11, it didn't delay me for long. Colleagues at the RPA cancer centre told me they thought I was mad to go, but I was determined. I took off two weeks later. Singapore Airlines was amazing as I was weighed down with two big suitcases packed with gowns and gloves and masks and colostomy bags (empty of course), and a whole heap of other equipment, too. It had been collected not only from RPA but from colleagues from all over Sydney who had heard about what I was doing. That included Tish Lancaster, who had whipped up a collection from Westmead Hospital. As I found myself inundated with equipment, Michael Boyer had to write a letter explaining not only why I was taking all this gear with me to Nepal, but also why I had in my possession a reasonably large quantity of generic pharmaceuticals. In those days Nepal didn't accept credit cards and nor did they have ATMs to get cash. Before leaving home I went to my local St George branch and asked for some travellers' cheques.

'Travellers' cheques? Where are you going?' they asked, so I told them I was heading off to Nepal for some voluntary work.

'What sort of voluntary work?' I was asked, so I told them.

'Would you be interested in taking some stuff up for the kids there?' they asked, and I said yes. So they donated small gifts to add to my already groaning array of medical gear: bags of balloons featuring the red and green dragon, colouring-in books, crayons, Textas, Vegemite, peanut butter and biscuits, plus those little packs of cheese and crackers. I ended up taking almost 100 kilos of medical gear and gifts for the children.

I had written to several airlines to see if they'd give me a free ticket because I was doing all this voluntarily, and while none would go quite that far, Singapore Airlines offered me my ticket at cost price, told me I could take as much stuff as I wanted, put me up in a hotel in Singapore, then flew me to Kathmandu in business class.

When I arrived at Tribhuvan International Airport in Kathmandu, I had to be met by a man with a van because we needed to lug all the equipment and gifts to Chitwan District, in west Nepal. Famous for its national park, its capital is Bharatpur, which is the largest city after Kathmandu, and while it is under 150 kilometres from the national capital, the roads were terrible and it took many hours for the van to get there. My destination was B.P. Koirala Memorial, a purpose-built cancer hospital run by the Nepal Cancer Relief Society, which was opened in honour of Bishweshwar Prasad Koirala, the first democratically elected Prime Minister of Nepal who died of throat cancer in 1982. Compared to the facilities in PNG, this hospital was far more advanced, although some of their chemotherapy equipment left a little to be desired.

I was there for four weeks in total and ran a morning course in the first week and an afternoon course in the second, so both sets of shift staff could attend the sessions. Unlike the courses in PNG, I had more nurses attend than doctors, so once there, I realised I would have to do a lot of writing to explain in detail to the local nurses, many of whom had only some degree of English, what I was demonstrating in the courses. Luckily, I was accompanied by Kate, another nurse who was a secretary in a former life. The hospital chairman offered us his office, so I'd sit with Kate and dictate notes while she typed. We wrote policy procedures, guidelines, job descriptions, appraisals, and a protocol book telling the staff how to give certain combinations of chemotherapy. Then I taught them how to prepare the cancer drugs, but not before we used a little outback ingenuity to make the equipment safer.

When I first saw the piece of equipment in the corner of the room where they were mixing the drugs, it looked more like a museum piece than modern medical equipment. It was an antique timber and glass hood with no safety venting and, as far as I could see, no other effective precautions were being taken in preparing these drugs. While I am the son of a carpenter, I did not inherit Dad's skills, so we grabbed a local engineer. We asked him to cut a hole in the top of the hood and place an accordion-type extraction pipe through it. This ran up to a vent on the wall near the ceiling and into a hole to the outside, so the fumes did not escape into the atmosphere inside the hospital. Then I offered all the donated white gowns, purple gloves and blue masks, because the staff didn't have anything remotely like the proper equipment. Finally, I proceeded to show the staff how to mix the drugs properly, transfer them and then administer them. I also evaluated the two wards and suggested that instead of two rooms full of beds, they have chairs for outpatients in one room and beds for sick patients who couldn't sit for long periods in the other.

The hospital also had a few machines, including a linear accelerator which is used for external beam radiation treatments for cancer patients, and a brachytherapy machine that places radioactive sources inside the patient to kill cancer cells and shrink tumours. Unlike PNG, the machines worked and there were radiation therapists to operate them, and they had a lot more knowledge and expertise than I did, as I was a chemotherapy nurse, not an expert in radiotherapy. However, I could see that they still lacked proper protocols and procedures and it was there that I could help.

As two white people in the middle of Nepal, we were considered a novelty, so the local kids used to come from around the district every afternoon after school to see us at the gate of the hospital compound. I'd come outside the house we were staying in and they'd be running down the street on the other side of the wall, repeatedly singing out, '*Ankal, ankal, ANKAL*,' or uncle in Nepalese. They were so exuberant, they'd wave and say hello, but that was the extent of our conversation. We knew nothing of their language and they knew nothing of ours, but it was very touching and they were so gorgeous. When they arrived one afternoon, we brought out the donated St George gifts and offered them balloons, colouring-in books and pencils. Their faces lit up, and they would puff out their cheeks, purse their lips and blow, indicating they wanted us to blow up the balloons for them. These are simple things that all children love, but some rarely see.

Nepal is one of the poorest countries in the world and has high levels of poverty, not that you'd know it from the smiles of the children, but their threadbare clothing and dirty faces were a giveaway. Only 10 per cent of the population were employed when we were there and there were no unemployment benefits, so how they survived I don't know. Lucky if they had a tin roof over their head, they didn't have much else at all, let alone fresh, running water. So one day, Kate and I decided to offer the kids a shower. There was a shower head that came out from a hole in the wall inside the compound, and while the water only trickled out, the kids stripped off to their undies and ran under the trickle and they loved it. I presume they'd never had a shower before and they ran in and out, over and over, laughing and joking with each other. While they were having fun, Kate and I washed all their clothes and put them on a flat roof to dry. It was quite hot so by the time they had finished playing under the water their clothes were dry and we dressed them and sent them home.

On the day of our departure, these kids came running down the street and grabbed at my legs and hugged me and wouldn't let go. They were all crying, too, because they'd heard that we were leaving. Their crying made me cry and it was all so sad. But we did a lot of good things while we were there. I'd love to go back to Nepal to see if all that we put in place at B.P. Koirala Memorial is still being used.

After finishing my work at Chitwan, I had some time off planned in Kathmandu with Daya, the director of nursing from B.P. Koirala Memorial. Daya, whose name means kindness or mercy, had taken three days off work, and on Sunday we drove back to Kathmandu with the hospital's medical oncologist. The trip along the narrow roads, through terraces of rice and fields of bright yellow mustard seed plants, was much more comfortable in a car than it had been in the van packed with medical supplies on the way up. Daya had organised for me to stay at a guesthouse, and while it was rustic, it had been modernised and had a much more comfortable bed than the one I'd had at the hospital in Chitwan. I still remember nodding off to sleep to the sound of Nepalese sarangi music drifting through my open window from the courtyard.

Each morning Daya would pick me up and we would then head to places she thought would be of interest. There were no tourists and the world was still stunned by 9/11. On our first full day, Daya took me on a guided tour via bus around Kathmandu before we headed off to lunch with her mum. I was invited into their house, an old, very basic place with two rooms where we sat on blocks of wood on the dirt floor in the kitchen and ate a lunch of rice and dahl with pickles and blanched wild greens with fresh, homemade roti presented on wooden boards. Daya spoke perfect English and she'd had some practice, having lived in Australia where she had completed much of her cancer training at the Peter MacCallum Cancer Centre in Melbourne. Her proud mother was listening intently as Daya interpreted what we had been up to over those past four weeks.

The next day we went to the Kathmandu Hospital where I met another oncologist and a head nurse and from there, we walked to the Fred Hollows Hospital nearby, named after the man I had treated almost a decade before. I was quite impressed. Like at B.P. Koirala Memorial, the facilities here weren't too bad at all compared to what I had seen in PNG. There was also a picture of Fred hanging over the entry, and it featured those distinctive magnifying glasses he wore while he worked. While I didn't see any eye operations, it was good to see Fred's legacy in action with all cataract surgeries now performed by local doctors.

On the third day, early in the morning, Daya and I headed to the Bagmati River where a crowd had gathered. It was the Vishwakarma Festival, where a representation of the god of craftsmen and architects is held aloft and paraded through the streets before both the idol and his followers are immersed in

159

the river to conclude the festival. Afterwards, Daya brought me back to the guesthouse where we said our farewells.

I had one last engagement before returning home. The simple meal with Daya and her mother a few days earlier was quite a contrast to the morning tea I was invited to at a palatial mansion that belonged to the parents of a fellow business class passenger who I'd sat beside on the way from Singapore to Kathmandu. She was Nepalese but lived in the US, and we'd got chatting on the flight. I'd told her all about what I was doing in Chitwan. 'When you are finished, you will have to come back to Kathmandu to join us for tea,' she said.

The compound was surrounded by a high fence. I rang a bell and the butler came to the gate, let me in and showed me to the front door where my fellow passenger and her parents greeted me. We had cups of tea and cake and I spoke with her parents who were interested in the work we were doing. These surroundings couldn't have been in greater contrast to those I had been immersed in over the past four weeks, but it was a lovely morning tea and I hope I was able to raise awareness about the work we were doing.

I got so much out of my trip to Nepal. While it's hard to get to these often remote destinations, it's even harder to leave because you grow so attached. I believe we made a real difference to the wonderful people and that special place.

18

CENTRE OF ATTENTION

A few months prior to my Nepal trip, early in 2001, I was with friends at a restaurant in Norton Street, Leichhardt, when my mobile started ringing. It was Frank Sartor, the then long-serving Lord Mayor of Sydney and later an MP in the NSW Parliament, known as the Bear Pit. While he could hold his own in parliament, on this occasion, Sartor was in dire straits and didn't know what to do. His partner Hephzibah Tintner had been diagnosed with a tumour on the tongue in 2000, just a few months after they had met. It was a Saturday night and she was in a great deal of pain, so I asked Frank what pain relief she had and when she had last taken it. I then asked him to increase the pain relief and also to make sure that she was comfortable staying at home rather than going to the hospital. He said he'd manage her care at home and took my advice on the pain relief. I called back later and he said the pain had lessened and she'd fallen asleep. I offered to visit if he needed my help.

She was already in palliative care by that stage and sadly Hephzibah died on 21 June 2001, at 30 years of age. Frank had also lost his mother to melanoma when he was just 16, so he had already joined the fight against cancer.

Our occupation of various floors at Gloucester House had become increasingly impractical, as it lacked patient privacy and was too small for the increasing number of patients who were being treated for cancer. By the early 2000s, the fight against cancer was on in earnest, driven not only by the medical profession but by politicians like Sartor, Sydney Lord Mayor from 1991–2003, who became the first chair of the Sydney Cancer Centre Foundation in 2001 before handing over both the lord mayoral chains and the foundation chair to Lucy Turnbull. He then moved into state politics and continued to be a champion for the cancer treatment cause. In those early years when he was mayor, Sartor had already met Jim Bishop and they had formed a joint alliance to raise $5 million in funding to add a new floor to Gloucester House, which was intended to be the heart of cancer treatment and the home of the Sydney Cancer Centre. The pair had also travelled to the US in 2002 to compare comprehensive cancer care centres at Johns Hopkins in Baltimore, Sloan Kettering in New York and the National Cancer Institute in Maryland.

When Bishop left to take charge of the newly created NSW Cancer Institute, Chris O'Brien and Michael Boyer, both of whom I had shown around as young medical students and registrars, also applied to fill the top Sydney Cancer Centre role. While I had returned to Australia and RPA in 1981, Chris – along with his wife Gail, toddler Adam and baby Juliette – followed my path to the UK, and also ended up at the Royal Marsden, where he continued his specialty in head and neck surgery and was also offered the position of honorary clinical fellow. While I had shared a flat in Earls Court – aka Kangaroo Valley – the O'Briens lived in Bernard Johnson House in East Finchley, in a self-contained flat provided for postgraduate couples and families like Chris's. After a year in London, Chris prepared to travel to the US, where he would secure the position of Head and Neck Oncology Fellow in the Department of Surgical Oncology at the University of Alabama. In contrast to the penury of the UK, which I also experienced, Chris's tenure in the US offered a reasonable wage and comfortable apartment in a complex which included swimming pools and tennis courts. It would be a few years before Chris would return 'home' to RPA, but when he did, in 1987, our paths would cross again.

By then, while I was already fully focused on oncology, Chris had returned as a very bright and very skilled head and neck surgeon. While we had some patients in common – those head and neck cancer patients who required chemotherapy and radiation therapy – it wasn't until well after that, when he and I were on various cancer committees, that we would work together closely again.

When Chris was eventually appointed director of the cancer centre, he also inherited a $5 million 'Raise the Roof' plan for Gloucester House, part of which included a fundraising campaign comprising the sale of tiny bricks, sold to donors for $100 each. It wasn't until Chris had been in the role for about 18 months that people started to say, 'Just putting another storey on the top of Gloucester House probably isn't a good idea for the new cancer centre.' The idea of an entirely new building started to gain traction.

In the planning phase, we had also looked at building out behind Gloucester House towards the Bosch Commons, a library in the grounds of Sydney University, and considered the Blackburn Building which is now part of the faculty of Medicine at Sydney University, but none of those building options was suitable. Chris became increasingly convinced that adding another floor to Gloucester House was not the way forward. As he wrote in his book, *Never Say Die*: 'I really did not think this was a good plan, in fact I thought it would be a waste of money'.

So a new building it was, but it would take a lot more than $5 million in mini-bricks to construct a brand new, state-of-the-art, purpose-built centre for the treatment of cancer, one to rival those that were emerging in the US and a first for NSW. It was during that period when Chris and I started to have a lot more to do with each other, and as we were fast running out of space in the heritage-listed Gloucester House, we both agreed the specialty of cancer – and the treatment of its patients – had to move on. As a state MP, Frank Sartor pushed the cause even harder, becoming Australia's first cancer minister with the added responsibility of forming the Cancer Institute NSW, which was eventually established in 2003. Sartor knew well the financial power and political might of lobby groups, especially after he took on the spin doctors when he introduced smoking bans in NSW pubs and clubs in 2004. But he had also secured a significant amount of cancer care funding from the private sector, including $750,000 from Ziggy Switkowski, then chief executive of Telstra.

By 2006, momentum had gathered and all interested medical parties met in the Kerry Packer Education Centre in RPA

164

to help organise a cancer research forum, and also arrange a dinner to celebrate the tenth anniversary of the Sydney Cancer Centre. I was on the organising team with Michael Boyer, Chris O'Brien and various other people. Even though we were all very busy, Chris piped up, 'What sort of coffee would you like, Keith?' and I said, 'Oh, I'll have a cappuccino, thanks.' So he went off himself and got me and everyone else a coffee and brought them back to the team. That's just the sort of thing he would do.

Our special guest at the forum was Ian Frazer, a Scottish-born Australian immunologist, and the founder, CEO and Director of Research of the Translational Research Institute. From his research at the University of Queensland, Ian, along with virologist and cancer researcher Jian Zhou, developed and patented the basic technology behind the HPV vaccine against cervical cancer. At our planning session, everyone was allocated jobs, and Chris asked if I'd mind picking up Ian from his hotel to bring him out to the forum. Chris knew that one of my pleasures was being able to pick up important people and spend a bit of quality time with them, one on one, while driving them around. I drove to the Hilton where Ian was staying and was delighted to ferry one of Australia's National Living Treasures, and a Florey Medallist to boot, back to the forum.

I didn't notice anything different about Chris that day and the forum went very well, along with the special dinner that followed. Chris had lots of charisma and people warmed to him as he warmed to them, no matter who they were, from politicians to royalty. He was able to talk to anyone and used that charm to ask then Liberal Prime Minister John Howard about funding the new cancer centre at RPA. But he wasn't going to put all his eggs in one basket, as there was a federal election coming up, so he started on Kevin Rudd and Labor as well. It didn't stop there, either! He also did the rounds of state government politicians, trying to scrounge money from wherever he could. On the federal side, Rudd had already promised that if Labor won the November 2007 election, he'd donate $100 million to the cause – with the proviso that the NSW Government should also kick in money. Instead, State Labor Premier Morris Iemma's cabinet committed to donating a property, the old Page Chest Pavilion opposite RPA. It had originally opened in 1957 as a tuberculosis treatment centre and over the decades had undergone several renovations and changes of use. In its latter years, it hosted various teams of cardiac specialists who went on to pioneer heart-lung bypass machinery use during surgery and hole-in-the-heart surgery, and it was also the place where Australian surgeons conducted the first successful fitting of a pacemaker. When Rudd came to power in November 2007, he made good on his promise and the Sydney Cancer Centre would soon become a reality.

Some of the people who would make the centre, later to be known as Chris O'Brien Lifehouse, possible, were those in the public eye who had been open about their diagnoses, or who used their platform to raise awareness and money for cancer research and treatment. Here are the stories of a few of those who made a lasting impression.

ANTHONY WARLOW (SURVIVOR)

It was 1992 and Anthony Warlow, Australian opera and musical theatre performer, was performing the lead role in *Phantom of the Opera* in Melbourne and was on an upward trajectory. He was pretty much approaching the peak of his career at that time and, apart from *Phantom*, was involved in pre-publicity for another big blockbuster, the revival of *Jesus Christ Superstar* in which he was to appear as Pilate. I first heard about Anthony's cancer from cardiologist Ian Wilcox. Ian and I had worked together when he did a term as a registrar in oncology at RPA, and we got on extremely well. Ian's wife's niece, Celia, was then married to Anthony. Ian paged me and I immediately called him back. 'We need an oncologist,' he said. 'This is confidential, but Anthony Warlow has a lump in his neck and we think it might be cancer.'

Anthony returned from Melbourne to his home in Sydney and was sent immediately to see Chris O'Brien because Chris was the best head and neck surgeon around. First of all, Anthony needed a firm diagnosis, which meant a CT scan, blood tests and biopsy to get a diagnosis of the cell type. The first biopsy revealed it was non-Hodgkin's lymphoma, and a highly aggressive one. Because it was in the lymphatic system – a network of vessels that transports a clear fluid called lymph around the body – Anthony needed to be 'staged' to see where it had spread. The lymphatic system includes the glands or lymph nodes that start at the neck and go all the way down to the groin. While this test is now redundant, Anthony had to have a lymphangiogram which involves taking a patient to nuclear medicine where they are injected with a blue dye in the webbing between the toes. The dye eventually works its way through the lymphatic system and the patient undergoes fluoroscopy to track the dye. After that test, Anthony then started undergoing a lot more tests that I was involved in or helped organise and which included lumbar punctures, bone marrow biopsies and other painful investigations.

Anthony would need 18 weeks of intravenous chemotherapy under oncologist Dr John Grygiel, so would come into the E9 Special Unit once every three weeks. There he was on a four-drug combination, three of which were given intravenously in the ward plus a steroid tablet which he had to take for five days after his chemotherapy. After that, he had to have intrathecal treatment, a process where they put a needle in the spinal canal and take out cerebral spinal fluid and inject chemotherapy into that space, a procedure he had to undergo twice a week. At the same time, he also had to have radiotherapy to his brain, which works as a prophylactic, because the type of lymphoma he had can spread to the brain and get into the cerebral spinal fluid, so this was the best treatment for cure along with systemic chemotherapy. Some of the drugs we used did not cross the blood-brain barrier, so this was used as extra protection.

After seeing his oncologist, Anthony was handed over to our chemotherapy team to coordinate the many hours of his treatment, so Anthony and I got to know each other very well. We discovered we had a lot of things in common and were very similar in many ways. His elder sister was a teaching nun at a church at Glebe. My elder sister was a nun. While he was brought up in Wollongong, he had a connection to Goulburn, as his father once had a photo studio in Auburn Street. I had also lived in Goulburn. We had our faith in common, too. He was a practising Roman Catholic, as was I. He's also great at telling jokes and is a great impersonator, taking off all sorts of accents, especially while telling a joke.

Understandably, his biggest concern was that the treatment would affect his singing voice, but he was always very positive and almost always happy. I was always trying to be positive, too,

168

and I wanted him to trust me and confide in me, just as I do all my patients. His was a very intense treatment regimen and included the loss of his blond locks, which have never grown back. As the chemotherapy unit was relatively small back then, I had time to be by Anthony's side for most of his chemotherapy treatment plus his intravenous treatment, which went on for a total of six months. After that, he came in for follow-up treatments and I was his first port of call whenever he arrived. If he had a problem, I was there to solve it.

When Anthony was given the all-clear after his successful treatment, he was very thankful. Even after John Grygiel left RPA and went to St Vincent's, Anthony wanted to stay at RPA because of the connection he had with me and the chemotherapy team. He felt comfortable there, so John sent him to Professor Graham Young to be followed up. This was once a month at first, then once every two months, then every three months, then six-monthly, then 12-monthly, and this went on for a couple of years after his treatment finished. But Anthony's career did get back on track and, despite some of the drugs being known to cause infertility, he and his wife Celia had a daughter, Phoebe.

After stepping back on stage, Anthony asked me to see his shows in Sydney where I was invited backstage for drinks. I also went down to Melbourne, to the Princess Theatre, where I saw him perform in *Phantom*, the staging of which was recreated specifically for Anthony after his recovery. He also praised his RPA treating team during a performance in *The Main Event* live concert tour at the Sydney Entertainment Centre, and it was backstage where I was lucky to meet his fellow performers, Olivia Newton-John and John Farnham. *The Main Event* was five years after his recovery and by then, he was being checked every 12 months. But if he did have a problem, needed some advice, or needed his bloods done, he'd give me a call or he would come in. Anthony always liked a cup of tea, so we'd sit, have a chat and catch up. If I was worried about anything in particular, I'd ring haematologist Graham Young, a Scotsman, and Graham would immediately say: 'I'll see him tomorrow' or 'I'll see him now, send him over', and he would see Anthony in the medical centre. As I said, Anthony was a great impersonator and after so many visits, he could do a great Graham Young impersonation, mimicking the Scottish burr so perfectly you'd think it was the real deal.

It's pretty handy having a world-class opera singer as a friend. When I was the local organising chair for the annual International Society of Nurses in Cancer Care, held at the old Sydney Convention Centre in 2004, I asked Anthony if he could help out in some way. He kindly volunteered to open the event. When a world-famous singer takes to the stage, be it a medical conference or *Phantom*, expect something dazzling. Anthony put on the most amazing performance and then closed the event with another brilliant solo performance. When we presented him with a gift of thanks, he told those thousands of nursing professionals attending our conference that he wouldn't be there, standing on that stage, if it wasn't for his treatment, and added that I had helped save his life. I still display a photo of us at that event which has pride of place on a mantle at my home.

Anthony doesn't need to see anyone now, me included, because he's so many, many years down the track from treatment, but he still telephones and texts. When he can, he now lives part of the year in New York, with his new partner, Amanda. But if he is in Sydney, we always meet in the city for coffee or go for lunch. It's a friendship I value highly.

MARC HUNTER (1953–1998)

The New Zealand–born lead singer and songwriter of the band Dragon lived life to the full and was well known for his hard living, having been a heroin addict for some time early in his career. When Marc was diagnosed with throat cancer in 1997, he was in his mid-40s, and I think he was clean at the time he was treated. Marc was very flamboyant, even when he was receiving chemo at Gloucester House while I was there. He used to parade around the ward in a blue and white Japanese kimono. I can still picture it now, especially when I hear his songs, 'April Sun in Cuba' and 'Are You Old Enough?', the band's hits of the 1970s and '80s, which I still have on tape. Marc was only 44 when he died on 17 July 1998.

JOHNNY WARREN (1943–2004)

In 2003, after smoking heavily for most of his life, soccer legend Johnny Warren publicly announced that he had been diagnosed with lung cancer. He was sent to Michael Boyer, and after further investigation it was decided Johnny needed chemotherapy. Michael asked me to get involved in his care. On his first visit, Michael ushered Johnny into the chemotherapy area of Gloucester Level 5. After being introduced, we went through what his treatment would entail and the side effects it would have. Then I showed him around the unit and asked if he had any questions. At one stage, Johnny had also been offered $50,000 by John Singleton to fund a trip and treatment at

MD Anderson Cancer Center in Houston, Texas, but he decided to be treated here.

Johnny was on a three-week cycle with carboplatin, used to slow or stop cancer cell growth, on day 1 and etoposide, which was given three days in a row, then he had a break for three weeks before he would start over again. He was a charismatic, jovial fellow, a bit like Chris O'Brien in that way. Gloucester 5 was open plan, so it looked a bit like an old-fashioned airport departure lounge. A patient would be sitting in a chair, hooked up to their bags of chemotherapy in the open ward, for two to three hours. Johnny's diagnosis was in the media by then, so everyone knew that the former Socceroo, TV host and author had lung cancer. He would come in for his treatment and we would try to give him some privacy. However, he would often be there in the open and passers-by immediately recognised him. He didn't seem to mind if he was approached by people for autographs.

Johnny did quite well on chemotherapy and didn't have a lot of side effects, and I think one of the reasons was because he had a very positive attitude. It makes a difference in how patients handle chemotherapy. If they are pessimistic and I tell them it might make you sick, they say: 'Well, I'll be sick because I always get sick. I go on an aeroplane and I get sick, I go on the Manly ferry and I get sick.' They sometimes talk themselves into being sick. But Johnny handled it quite well.

While I didn't follow soccer very closely, I knew his team was St George FC and, coincidentally, my father had played for the same team. While Johnny had played for them from 1963–64, my dad had taken to the field in the 1920s when he had lived in Sydney. I now really regret that when we had to clear out the old post office, shop and petrol station at Cullerin, we threw out all of Dad's old team photos and the St George premiership cups he'd had. But Johnny and I had that rapport about St George, and we chatted a bit about it, among other things, when I checked in on him during his treatments.

During that period Johnny had some time when he was disease-free, so he put his energy into a fundraising event for the Sydney Cancer Centre, which at the time was run by Jim Bishop. Johnny's motivation was twofold: number one was that he wanted to do something for us at the centre, and number two, he knew funding for all types of cancers was not especially good – and at that particular time we were also trying to raise money to expand the unit. Johnny had lots of connections and plenty of friends, plus there were all of us at RPA who were involved in his care, and we were invited too. It was held at Le Montage, a waterfront venue in Leichhardt, and was a full house with well-known sports journalist Les Murray hosting the big event in the ballroom. Unfortunately, Johnny relapsed not long after.

With shortness of breath and in a lot of pain, the decision was made to go down the path of palliative care at Prince Alfred, so I'd often duck up to see Johnny on Level 7 East in the new Clinical Services block where the oncology inpatients were. He was asked where he would like to continue his treatment and he decided he wanted to be at home in Jamberoo on the NSW south coast. But his palliative care away from RPA was brief and he died soon after, on 6 November 2004. NSW Premier at the time, Bob Carr, announced that Johnny would be provided with a state funeral at St Andrew's, next to Sydney Town Hall, marking the first time such an event was offered to a sporting figure. In 2017, Murray also succumbed to cancer and was given the same honour.

'Johnny Warren was a great Australian,' Mr Carr said in a statement. 'He was Mr Football – the man with vision and passion for developing the "world game" in Australia.'

It was the first and only time that I've ever been formally invited to a funeral via written invitation, and I attended along with Michael Boyer and another nurse, Caroline, from the Sydney Cancer Centre, who Johnny had warmed to.

As much as I try to resist giving people special treatment, it is hard not to treat them differently when they are personalities or friends or relatives of friends. When Michael Boyer's brother David was diagnosed with colon cancer, Michael said to me, 'Keith, I may need your help.' So I was there when David started treatment at Gloucester House and I was there when he had his last treatment at Lifehouse when it opened in 2013. It's difficult to separate those patients who you are closely connected to in some way, as they get to know you a bit more and have a tendency to become reliant on you as a nurse. Patients also become accustomed to the way you do things, too, which offers them a sense of comfort and familiarity. If someone else was put in charge of their treatment, they'd say: 'Oh, but Keith puts the cannula in this way', or 'You're gonna put the cannula in there? Keith doesn't put it there!' But if you gave everyone special treatment you wouldn't get all your work done. In the end, as I always said, 'We work as a team' – sometimes you might get a different nurse, but we are all team players in the game. Johnny would have understood that.

CELEBRITY SUPPORTER JENNIFER HAWKINS

Since being crowned Miss Universe, Jennifer Hawkins has been using her high profile to make a difference, donating to many of the cancer charities I have been involved in, including Sydney Cancer Foundation and CanTeen. While Jennifer didn't have cancer, it is a cause that is close to her heart as, unfortunately, her mother was diagnosed with kidney cancer and underwent surgery in Newcastle to remove a kidney in 2015. Before, during and after treatment, I always respect the privacy of the patient and their family and rarely, if ever, do I have a photo taken with anyone on a ward. But one I treasure is of Jennifer and her then fiancé Jake Wall – they are now married and have two children – on a tour of the Sydney Cancer Centre after she made one of her generous financial contributions. This was while she was still the reigning Miss Universe, in 2004.

19

FILLING THE GAPS

As a surgeon, Chris O'Brien adhered to a model of care in which he only engaged clinical nurse consultants (CNCs) who had specialist knowledge and a specific understanding of the treatment of patients with that particular illness which, in his case, was head and neck cancers. While his CNCs later became nurse practitioners, my specialty was filling in the gaps where there wasn't a specialist CNC, which included quite a few areas in the early days such as sarcoma, lung cancer and testicular cancers. In contrast, we had specific breast cancer nurses and in the latter years, the McGrath Foundation has been able to financially support as many as 60–80 of them.

As I was one of the few male CNCs, I was called on quite a lot for cases of boys and men affected by testicular cancer because, as I've mentioned, I've found men relate a lot better to another man when they are talking about fertility, sperm banking, sexual function and the possibility of losing a testicle.

In those earlier days, we also had social workers who a patient could talk to if they had relationship problems or issues arising from their treatment. But we didn't have that many psychologists, so I became involved there as well. Things are a lot better now, as the model of care is to have a nurse attached to each particular diagnosis, be it lung cancer, breast cancer, upper or lower gastrointestinal cancer, sarcoma, head and neck cancer or melanoma – and there are now specialised nurses in each of these areas.

While I enjoyed being a clinical nurse consultant, I was also thinking about taking the next step to become a nurse practitioner. The process was a long one – it would end up taking me almost a decade. In the mid-1990s, Martin Tattersall and Michael Boyer applied to the NSW Department of Health to trial a nurse practitioner in cancer care – and their candidate was me. The application was open to all specialities, but only about ten positions would be funded. Unfortunately, our first attempt was unsuccessful and the funding went to midwifery services for much-needed midwives in rural and remote areas, and to nurses in A&E. By the time 2004 came around, the oncology department was based at Gloucester House, and while there was no funding for nurse practitioners, these specialist roles were being established elsewhere throughout the country.

I knew that in my time, cancer treatments, technology and therapies had developed and changed dramatically, and as a registered nurse, I could look and enquire and ask what suited a patient best, and conduct numerous patient satisfaction surveys. It was this knowledge and experience that I wanted to use to improve patient outcomes. I was already considered an advanced practice nurse with many years of experience, but

I still had to ask a doctor to request a blood test for a patient, to order patient fluids or pain relief medication. If an intern could do this straight out of medical school, with my three decades of cancer treatment, why couldn't I? If I was authorised as a specialist cancer nurse practitioner, however, I would be able to 'prescribe, order and refer'. In other words: prescribe medication or pain relief, order blood tests, send patients off to radiology for CT scans and X-rays or refer patients to other specialists within my scope of practice – which in my case was oncology. Another reason why a cancer nurse practitioner would be valuable was that nurses conduct a high proportion of the follow-up check-ups of survivors and monitor their progress. A doctor might see a new patient for one or two hours initially, with regular follow ups, but I would sometimes see that same patient more often, and frequently over a longer period of time, plus I've seen different cancers and patient survival rates and I've observed, firsthand, the varying drug regimens used.

Armed with that belief, in 2004 I embarked once again on the process of becoming a cancer nurse practitioner. In those days, there were two pathways to becoming a CNP. The first was to have 5000 hours at an advanced practice level plus a Masters degree. The second, my preferred pathway, was to have 5000 hours at an advanced practice level, proof of qualifications, plus any research you had been involved in and a copy of any published works, plus any awards. In addition, you were required to supply four referees to support your application, and a detailed case study of a patient which covered five areas to demonstrate where your skills as a CNP would be able to be utilised. Those five areas were the clinical manifestation and physical description of the cancer, mode of spread of the cancer, treatment options, various investigations such as tumour markers and describing and understanding what they meant, plus the psychosocial needs of the patient. Accompanying the portfolio was another scope of practice document specifying all the medications I would be allowed to prescribe. All of this had to be bundled up into a portfolio and in the end, my 200 plus–page document was about the thickness of a dictionary and weighed about 1.5 kilograms. It was then submitted to the Nurses Registration Board, and after some to-ing and fro-ing, I had to appear before a panel and then make a second appearance to answer a few more questions.

In December 2006 I received notification that my application had been successful.

20

A PRINCE AMONG PATIENTS

DOUGLAS YORATH (1971–2005)

I've touched a lot of lives in my career and must have treated around 30,000–40,000 patients. And like I've said, you treat them all the same, but I guess it's just human nature that you warm to some people more than others. There are various degrees of friendship and, of course, there are degrees of love as well. I'd been away on holiday when 32-year-old Doug Yorath was first sent to us at RPA. He had sarcoma, cancer that starts in tissue such as bone or muscle, and he'd already had a fore-quarter amputation – which is the removal of the whole shoulder and arm. Martin Tattersall, whose specialty was sarcomas among other things, was his oncologist, and Doug had already started his chemotherapy. On this particular Tuesday, we were in Gloucester 5 and Martin came in just after lunchtime.

'Keith,' he said, 'I'm seeing a young fellow today. His name is Doug and I want you to be involved in his care, so would you have a minute to meet him?'

181

At the time there were no specialist CNCs for sarcomas, and I wasn't yet a cancer nurse practitioner, but Martin wanted me, as a CNC who specialised in oncology and chemotherapy, to help with Doug's case. Martin brought him in to meet me, introduced us, then left us together to have a long discussion about treatment.

Doug was one of the most amazing young men I've ever come across. He had a sort of aura about him. Even though he only had one arm and one hand, he could operate almost as normal. He could drive a car, get dressed on his own, and insisted on doing most things for himself. He had a practical way of looking at things. He used to wear riding boots so he could pull the strap up, so he didn't have to tie up shoelaces. I remember saying to him, just the once, 'Do you want me to put on your boots for you?' and he said: 'No, I can do it.' It was clear he didn't want my help with simple things like that. Part of his can-do attitude had to do with his being an occupational health and safety officer. It wasn't until much later in the piece that I found out he had also trained as a nurse. It's not the main reason why I think we got on, but we did get on extremely well and that may have been part of it. Doug could relate to me and I could relate to him, and he could talk to me about anything.

Unfortunately, Doug already had metastatic disease when I met him, which is when cancer cells spread to new areas of the body, so he was on treatment to try to improve his quality of life and lengthen it as much as possible. Despite his treatment, he continued to live in his own apartment, but his father Don was always at the hospital by his side when he came in for treatment. I also met Doug's mother and sister, and was introduced to some of his friends, too, and we all became quite close.

Doug and I used to talk a lot in the days and weeks that followed, and it was occasionally about faith or his family or his work. During the course of one conversation, he said to me: 'Oh, you know my pastor.' I said, 'Who's that?' It turned out that all the time I'd known him, Doug had been attending the Presbyterian church in Drummoyne, just down the road from my house. Personally, I always enjoyed having conversations with patients who had some form of religious faith and often found a common avenue of communication with them.

It was around this time we were told that His Royal Highness The Prince of Wales wanted to visit a cancer centre while he was on his whistle-stop tour of Sydney. I was approached by Chris O'Brien, then the director of the Sydney Cancer Centre, to organise a group of patients to meet Prince Charles at the hospital named after his forebear. I chose Doug Yorath as one of four patients and their relatives who agreed to meet the prince and they all had to sign media consent forms and undergo security checks before the big day. The hospital was visited by various security details, including the Federal Police and the prince's people. On the day of Prince Charles's visit in March 2005, security came and completed another sweep of the unit before HRH was due to arrive at 2.30 pm.

We had to separate the select group of four, including Doug, from the rest of the patients, who were all moved to the back of the ward on Gloucester 5. The prince's large entourage arrived, including Sydney Cancer Centre director Chris O'Brien, Health Minister Morris Iemma, NSW Premier Bob Carr and RPA's general manager. Just before Prince Charles entered the room, I was briefed by his aide. I was told I could shake the prince's hand when introduced, then walk on the prince's left-hand side as we made our way along the ward. But I wasn't allowed to touch the royal person – although I absent-mindedly did on two occasions but fortunately didn't get into any trouble. I introduced His Royal Highness to Doug, Doug's parents, plus the other three patients and their families. Doug looked great on the day. He used to wear long-sleeved shirts and had a prosthesis to give him the appearance of a shoulder, but had to tuck the sleeve up as he didn't have an arm or a hand. The visit was well timed as it was a Friday afternoon and the unit wasn't too busy, and we had limited the number of treatments scheduled that afternoon. The prince was on a tight schedule, but nevertheless, after he'd greeted the four selected patients and their families, he noticed the cluster of remaining patients squeezed up the back of the ward peering down.

'Keith,' Prince Charles said to me, 'what about all those other people up there? I can't not meet them.'

With an urgent whisper to attendant staff, we got more consent forms to the other patients who quickly filled them out. Hands behind his back, Prince Charles then strolled over to the rest of the eager patients on the ward that day and met every single one, spending quite a few minutes with each, talking about their treatment. What impressed me most was that he would have an informed discussion with each of them. One patient was having a blood transfusion and while she wasn't one of the two women who we had earlier organised, the prince knew her particular treatment and spoke to her about it. He was well briefed overall and was able to hold a conversation on cancer, chemotherapy and blood transfusions and commented on how important it was to donate blood. He probably stayed on the ward for about 40 minutes before he was driven to the airport and boarded a plane to Canberra. The Prince of Wales left a very positive feeling at our cancer centre at RPA that day, and it was an uplifting occasion for both patients and staff.

Shortly after the royal visit, Doug underwent surgery to remove a secondary brain tumour that had been preventing him from talking. On rounds the morning after his surgery, Doug surprised surgeon Michael Besser and his team by demonstrating how quickly and completely he had recovered. The surprises for the surgical team continued when, not long after returning to live with his parents, Doug phoned Professor Besser's office to ask whether, so soon after the surgery, he would permit Doug to go for a joy flight in a helicopter piloted by Doug's cousin, Brenton. It was Doug's parents' anxiety that persuaded him not to accept the offer. It was just a few weeks after the royal visit and Doug's subsequent neurosurgery when Doug's father Don rang me.

'Doug's not doing very well and I'm wondering if I could bring him in?' Don said. I told Don to take Doug straight into the chemotherapy unit at Gloucester 5 where I liked to deal with most of my patients if I could, rather than having them admitted through RPA Emergency. Doug looked terrible when he arrived. He was having a lot of difficulty breathing, was in great discomfort and had cyanosis, a blue discolouration around the mouth which indicates a lack of oxygen.

'Doug, I think you might have some fluid on the lung,' I told him. 'It's called pleural effusion. I'm going to send you for an X-ray.'

As he was so unwell, Doug was immediately put on oxygen. I called the X-ray department and explained the circumstances, then went down with Doug to the main hospital. After his

X-ray, I brought him back to the unit and contacted Professor Tattersall, confirming that Doug had a pleural effusion as suspected, was most unwell and needed to be admitted. Doug's total lung capacity was about 30 per cent, so you could understand why he was finding it so difficult to breathe. Even though I was a CNC, I couldn't admit a patient back then and needed Professor Tattersall to do it. Prof also approved his registrar to conduct a pleural tap, so we were able to find a private room for Doug in the chemotherapy unit and aspirate the pleural effusion, removing most of the fluid affecting one lung. To do this, a special needle called a stiletto is inserted into the back, between a couple of ribs, then into the pleural space between the lung and the pleura, the outside membrane where the fluid builds up. The pleural tap kit comes with a tube connecting it to an underwater sealed drain which effectively sucks out the fluid, or you can slowly draw the fluid off with a syringe via a three-way valve, as we did in this case. After removing a significant amount of fluid, Doug was a bit more comfortable. Although he had been treated as an outpatient for most of his treatment, and he had done very well, you could now take one look at him and know he didn't have much time left.

'Doug, I think we're going to need to admit you into the hospital. As much as you don't like being in hospital, I don't think I can manage all this with you as an outpatient,' I said. He agreed, but you could see a little bit of fear in his face and he wasn't a very good colour. I took him up to the ward and explained I couldn't stay with him very long as I had to get back to the chemotherapy unit, but that I would return later. Doug was so breathless and distressed at that point that he couldn't talk but I believe your eyes talk for you in these situations, and I had been there before. Doug was able to communicate to me that he wanted me to return. After finishing at the chemotherapy unit, I returned to Doug's side and spent just over an hour chatting with him and his family who had arrived to be by his bedside. He couldn't lie flat by then and had to sit up in bed to ease the pressure on his lungs and help with his breathing. We raised the bed and put a lot of pillows around him and I gave him morphine to help with his respiratory difficulties. I also administered midazolam, which helps patients relax. We made sure he was as comfortable as he could be and I continued to chat with him and his family.

'Doug, I'm just going to go home for a bit of dinner, but if you want me to come back, I will,' I said. This was directed as much at Doug's parents as it was to him because you just don't know exactly how much a patient can understand or can hear at this late stage of their life, drifting in and out of consciousness, as hearing is the last sense to go.

I arrived home and, true to form, the front door of my neighbours' place opened, and there were Dante and Anna offering me a home-cooked dinner. I can't remember what they had cooked for me that night but, as always, it was delicious and saved me from preparing a meal. I ate it silently and had just put the television on to relax, exhausted from the long day, when the phone rang. It was Terrence, one of the nurses from the ward.

'Keith, can you come back? Doug's parents want you here as Doug's quite distressed.'

I dashed back to RPA and was quite shocked to hear Doug gasping for air even before I had entered the ward. I entered his room, stood by his bedside and gently rubbed his back.

'Doug, it's OK to let go now,' I told him. Then, knowing that Doug was a man of faith, I said, 'Our Lord has got your room ready for you and you can let go and go to your Maker,' hoping this would offer him some comfort. 'Do you want me to go or to stay with you?' I said, and Doug indicated he wanted me to stay. I remained with the family until just after midnight when Doug drew his last breath. It probably took almost two hours for him to go, and he was still battling up to his last half hour. It wasn't what I would call a peaceful death and it was quite hard for all of us who were there with him – his parents, sister and me. Although I wasn't a family member and I'd only known him for a relatively short time in his life, I was honoured that he wanted me to be there with him. What a huge privilege it was for me to be at his bedside during those final moments.

Doug passed away on 4 May, not long after that royal visit. But a sense of peace came over me soon after his death and in the days that followed, and I felt strongly that I wanted to attend his funeral. But you can't just go to a funeral when you are rostered on for hospital duty. As a senior nurse, I had to ask my immediate boss for the day off. Then Don rang me before the funeral: 'Keith, we would like you to sit with us.'

It was quite an honour to sit with his family in the front row of Drummoyne Presbyterian Church, just a few hundred metres from my house, to say one last goodbye to a young man I hardly knew in the beginning but got to know very well at the end during his many months of treatment. Don was kind enough to mention me in his eulogy.

I particularly want to mention Keith Cox (sitting with us today), clinical nurse consultant, whose care and attention throughout

Doug's treatment at RPA was of inestimable help to Doug and to us in coping with his treatment and managing the consequences. Keith promised Doug he would 'travel the road' with him. He really did, right to the end at ten minutes past midnight that last day.

It was a lovely service and a fitting closure to Doug's earthly life. They had a lot of singing and beautiful music, as Doug liked his music, and he liked that Presbyterian church too and felt very bonded to it. After the service, the rector and assistant priest at his parents' Anglican church, Reverend Keith Dalby and Reverend John Spooner, accompanied Doug's body to the crematorium. Meanwhile, family and friends spent time at the wake reminiscing about the life of this amazing young man.

21

GOD! CHRIS LOOKS SO TIRED

CHRIS O'BRIEN (1952–2009)

While he was busy running around the country, trying to raise funds, sitting on various boards, conducting surgeries and seeing patients, I noticed Chris O'Brien was starting to look very pale. On one particular Friday in November 2006, we were on Level 5, where the chemotherapy and the clinics were. I saw Chris – mobile phone stuck to his ear as usual – going down in the lift with Michael Boyer. I looked in as the doors started closing and said hello to them both. Michael said 'Hi' back but Chris continued with his phone conversation. I thought, *God! Chris looks so tired. He doesn't look well at all.* The following Monday, I was flying to Melbourne for an annual medical conference on cancer and was at Sydney Airport ready to board my flight when Michael rang me. It was a one-sided conversation that I'll never forget. 'Keith, I don't think you know yet,' he said, 'but Chris O'Brien has been admitted to hospital and he's got a brain tumour.'

I had my boarding pass in my hand, ready to get on the flight, but had to step back in shock. I just started crying and, of course, I didn't know anyone around me, they were all strangers. There I was, about to fly to Melbourne to attend meetings and listen to lectures about cancer, when I was told that Australia's leading head and neck surgeon had a malignant brain tumour. Michael went on to say that he had to take over from Chris, as he was second in charge, and he would be running everything while they worked out what the prognosis was for Chris.

The next few days in Melbourne were a blur; it was hard to focus on my medical lectures and meetings. Chris's diagnosis was the talk of the medical conference. Everyone knew, not just the cancer teams – everyone. One reason was that by then, Chris was a familiar face on the Channel 9 series *RPA*, in which he had appeared since Series 2 in 1996.

On the Wednesday of that week, four days after his initial diagnosis and two days after his discharge following a course of drugs to reduce the swelling to his brain, Chris and his wife Gail met Professor Michael Besser to discuss the scans and the ideal treatment. Surgery was planned for the following Sunday where they would attempt to remove the tumour. When pathology studied the biopsy, they discovered it was a glioblastoma multiforme or GBM, the fast-growing glioma that develops from star-shaped glial cells (called astrocytes and oligodendrocytes) that support the health of the nerve cells within the brain. GBMs are the most invasive type of glial tumours, rapidly growing and commonly spreading into nearby brain tissue. They are like an octopus with tentacles that burrow into the brain and are very difficult to get out. But I was always surprised by how quickly some patients recover from brain surgery, none more so than Chris, who was awake and alert soon after his operation.

Later, Chris had radiotherapy in conjunction with an oral chemotherapy drug called temozolomide, and it was at this stage that I became involved in his care. Radiotherapy was administered Monday to Friday in an RPA building in Salisbury Road, and Chris's oral chemotherapy was taken continuously throughout the radiotherapy treatment. While both Gail and Chris knew that they could contact me anytime for help or advice, I would often pop over to see them in the radiotherapy building to make sure they were both OK, and I'd sit with Gail as Chris lay flat out on a bed in the lead-lined radiotherapy room undergoing treatment. The drug temozolomide, also known as Temodar, often makes patients feel nauseous, as does radiotherapy, so patients often throw up a lot, which limits the effectiveness of the drugs. So Chris was on an antiemetic to decrease nausea, and also on dexamethasone, a steroid that is part of a combination of anti-sickness drugs that are used for those patients with cerebral oedema, a brain tumour or who are having cerebral radiotherapy.

While he had these first-line treatments, sadly Chris's cancer progressed and he sought other options, including surgery and carboplatin, an intravenously administered drug with fewer side effects than cisplatin. An anti-sickness medication is administered first, then the carboplatin is administered in a 500-millilitre bag of fluid. While I had a broader role as an oncology-chemotherapy nurse consultant, I would occasionally be involved in cannulation and the administration of Chris's drug treatment. My specialty is symptom management, so controlling vomiting, dehydration and fatigue was an important part of Chris's treatment. I'd also help him overcome other ongoing side effects and fatigue which came as a result of the carboplatin. During this time Chris was also investigating alternative therapies and sought a second opinion. In addition, he contacted renowned brain surgeon Charlie Teo and later went to another brain cancer specialist at Royal North Shore Hospital. He had an alternative trial drug treatment there, too. As Chris was a head and neck surgeon, he knew the prognosis was not good, so he was willing to try anything to beat the cancer that was killing him.

A TV crew had been a familiar sight at RPA and I had often shown a cameraman, sound assistant and producer through the cancer wards. They could also often be seen trailing Chris on his rounds while he spoke with various patients, doctors and nurses. By 2007, and then in its 13th series, *RPA* had become Australia's longest-running reality TV series. Little did we know that Chris would be on the other side of the patient–doctor discussion of an episode of *RPA* in Series 14. He would also be followed by a *60 Minutes* crew and then reporter Peter Overton, plus have newspaper features written about his cancer battle. Chris was such a well-known face by then that he was often approached in the middle of his IV treatment in the old chemotherapy unit at Gloucester House 5. Staff, patients and colleagues would walk past, stop and say hi, or would have a chat while he sat having his chemotherapy. The unit had 22 chairs and five beds in total, which included a curtained-off four-bedded bay and a fully curtained-off small, single room at the end of the ward. In it was a hospital bed in front of a window, next to a chest-high wall, which offered some privacy. It was also the room where we put patients whose treatment we wanted to observe if they had adverse effects. It was the place where cricket commentator Tony Greig had been treated some years earlier and the room where Chris would end up too, in an attempt to give him some peace and quiet during his treatment.

Despite Chris's intensive treatment and the attention he was getting, we still spoke a lot about the proposed Sydney Cancer Centre, the name of which would later change to Lifehouse. Despite his illness, it was still at the forefront of his very active mind. Chris was focused on creating a comprehensive cancer treatment centre where patients could receive all forms of treatment, from the traditional to the complementary. He wanted this to include relaxation therapy, acupuncture and exercise physiology along with meditation and the advice of a dietician, all the therapies he had been seeking himself. Chris continued to work in the political lobbying space too, including attending one fundraising launch at Government House where he was so weak, his son Adam had to help him on stage to speak.

Very sadly he soon relapsed and despite further surgery under the hand of Charlie Teo, Chris was all too soon at the palliative care stage. His family's plan had been for him to die at his Hunters Hill home, surrounded by loved ones. I helped where I could and became involved in Chris's care, to try to keep him home and grant the family's wish.

One Friday morning in May 2009, Gail called me to say Chris was in a terrible state so I drove over to their house. When I arrived, Chris had been vomiting all night and was looking very weak. If a patient is vomiting, they don't absorb their oral medication very well, be it pain relief or cancer medication, and as he had all these debilitating symptoms I said to Gail, 'Look, we have to get him to hospital, straight away.'

We decided not to wait for an ambulance, so I helped get Chris in the car, telling Gail I would leave my car at their house and come in with them to RPA to help arrange his admission. Once we arrived at the hospital, we rehydrated him and kept him on IV, medication and other fluids until he improved enough over a couple of days to return to the family home.

But just a few weeks later, Gail called again and said the family was bringing him back into RPA because he was so unwell. While the nearest hospital to their home would have been Royal North Shore, Chris's family wanted him to be admitted to RPA, so we arranged for the ambulance to bring him in to Gloucester House. After they all arrived, the ambulance officers and I transferred Chris into a hospital bed on Level 5, where we got his pain under control. Michael Boyer was away at the time so Lisa Horvath (now head of medical oncology at Lifehouse) was looking after Michael's patients. While Chris was given morphine and anti-sickness drugs and made more comfortable, Lisa had to tell the family that there was not a lot more that could be done. We could only keep him comfortable. 'This is it, really,' she said.

While arrangements were made for his readmission, Chris's son James and I wheeled the virtually unconscious Chris up to E10 ward and into a private room. His condition failed to improve and the next day, I received a call from the CEO of RPA. 'The Prime Minister, Kevin Rudd, wants to come and say goodbye to Chris O'Brien,' she said. The PM was about to jump on a flight from Canberra and I was told a security officer would call me to confirm his arrival at Mascot and give me his expected arrival time at RPA. The CEO said that because it was not an official visit, she wanted me to personally meet the PM at the rear entrance then show him up to Chris's room, via the staff lifts. Not many people were about, as it was early evening, so few noticed the COMCAR vehicle roll up to the entrance of RPA in Gloucester Drive. The PM stepped out of the car, without a security detail in sight, and offered me his hand. 'Kevin,' he said, and I shook his hand and introduced myself.

We took a service lift together to Level 10 and to the room where Chris was with his immediate and extended family. We all knew he didn't have many hours left. I must say Kevin was fantastic, holding Chris's hand and spending a few moments with him in quiet contemplation before the nurses needed to tend to their patient. So we left them to their work. Kevin and I went out for a short while but soon returned to Chris's bedside where his immediate family – Gail, James, Juliette and Adam – were with him. The PM had some paperwork with him and spoke quietly to Chris in his bed: 'Chris, I'm giving you an Order of Australia,' he said, and he began to read out the citation for an AO.

Those of us in the room believe Chris knew what was happening as there were some small changes in his facial movement, and Kevin also said later that Chris had squeezed his hand. Kevin Rudd had got to know the family quite well over the two-and-a-half years of Chris's diagnosis, so there were many hugs and kisses and tears in the room that evening. After reading the citation, the PM said goodbye to the O'Brien family and left Chris's bedside. I led him to a private room and asked him, 'How are you, Kevin?'

'I feel like shit,' he said, close to tears. He revealed that he had not seen anyone that close to death before. As nurses, we are often close to the dying. There are many different types of death, too. It's not that we become immune to it, but we do become accustomed to it, and we build up coping mechanisms to deal with it. Some people take a long time to die, others die suddenly, so I see it all the time and this wasn't new to me. But for most people it's a new and confronting experience. I looked at the PM and asked if there was anything I could do. 'Just sit with me for a while,' he said as he composed himself before flying back to a parliamentary sitting in Canberra that night. The PM must have arrived back in Canberra about 9.30 pm, but only a few hours after that, just before midnight on 4 June 2009, Chris O'Brien AO passed away.

The PM returned to attend Mass with the O'Briens at their local church, Villa Maria in Hunters Hill. In addition he offered the family a state funeral for Chris, which Gail accepted. Gail met parish priest Father Kevin Bates to make funeral arrangements, not for a simple ceremony as originally planned but a major event at St Mary's Cathedral, which would be attended by hundreds of mourners including extended family, dignitaries, medical colleagues and former patients. I went to the O'Briens' house to see the family and Father Kevin and it was agreed that I would assist at the funeral as an acolyte, a role I was familiar with as I had been assisting at my local church services at St Mark's in Drummoyne since 1992.

On the day of Chris's funeral, 11 June 2009, dressed in my white acolyte robe which is called an alb, I hugged each of the family members as they took their seats. Father Kevin welcomed everyone and moved around the casket, blessing it and sprinkling it with holy water. I approached each of the eulogists – surgeon Mark Malouf, Michael Boyer, family friend and BridgeClimb founder Paul Cave, and Kevin Rudd – in order of the book of service, and took them up to the lectern where they completed their eulogies, after which I returned them to their seat. St Mary's convention usually permits only one eulogy, but Gail insisted on the four that she and Chris had agreed on, and Cardinal George Pell eventually relented. Towards the end of the service, I took Gail and Juliette up to the lectern together, where they spoke, one at a time.

At the end of the service, when the coffin was being put in the hearse, I was with Juliette and her brother James, still in my white robe, when a newspaper photographer took an image of me with my arms around them both. It appeared the following day, mistakenly identifying me as one of the clergy. I returned to the sacristy to change out of my alb and meet with Michael Boyer and his wife Fran. We all went to the Northern Suburbs Crematorium together where Father Kevin offered a short service and commended Chris's spirit to God. Family friend and neighbour Col Joye took up his ukulele and sang 'Somewhere Over the Rainbow' as Chris's coffin disappeared.

Afterwards, we returned to town and the wake, which was being held in Guillaume, then a restaurant under a sail of the Sydney Opera House and run by Guillaume Brahimi, a good friend of the O'Briens. This hatted chef had offered Chris and his family home-cooked meals and special treats during Chris's illness and the Brahimi children, Constance and Honor, had brought the offertory to the altar during the funeral service. At the wake, Kevin Rudd approached Gail who was sitting by herself on a long curved seat inside the cavernous restaurant. As Juliette O'Brien recounts in *This Is Gail*, the memoir she wrote about her mother:

'I want to ask your permission for something, Gail. Lifehouse should be named after Chris. Would you give your permission for it to be the Chris O'Brien cancer centre?'

'Yes, of course,' she told the Prime Minister, instantly thrilled at the thought of Chris's name living on in bricks and mortar, a glorious testament to what he had lived for. Kevin Rudd put his arms around her then took the microphone.

'I have just been chatting with Gail. She has agreed to have Lifehouse named after Chris. From now on it will be known as the Chris O'Brien cancer centre at RPA.'

Cheers erupted as the crowd agreed it was right.

Michael Boyer and I were very much on the same page about Chris's vision for a new cancer centre but he died a year before we pulled down the old Pavilion building and Lifehouse rose in its place. After Chris's death, and thanks to his foresight, early fundraising and political pressure, the therapy space that he envisioned now exists at Lifehouse in the form of the LivingRoom, and features adjunct consulting rooms, a kitchen, gym and prayer rooms overlooking the Tree of Life, which is a void in the building planted with species such as native livistona palms, luminous cyathea and green tree ferns. While our shared vision has come to life and has now celebrated almost a decade of care, many of those original ideas and much of the philosophy came from Chris. When Lifehouse officially opened, I thought, *This is stuff that we all talked about and we've worked on for many years*. For all of us who were involved, Lifehouse was a dream come true.

22

NURSING IN THE NEIGHBOURHOOD

ANNA FERZOCO (1934–2017)

When she was in her late 70s, Anna Ferzoco, my neighbour and second mother, developed uterine sarcoma, a rare-ish cancer that forms in bone or connective tissue. We treat this particular cancer as we would any soft tissue sarcoma, which is with chemotherapy drugs, not the drugs normally used in the treatment of uterine cancer. Anna had surgery to remove the sarcoma at RPA, then would have chemotherapy and radiotherapy in Lifehouse, which had not long opened. So my neighbour became my patient.

Initially, Anna had a good response post-surgery but still needed radiotherapy and chemotherapy. If she needed a check-up and had to have her bloods done, I'd take her in to work with me then I'd ring Dante when she was finished and he would drive over and pick her up. I made sure I organised all her morning appointments so they would coincide with my schedule. While Anna had a really good response after both therapies, she did have a few problems. She wouldn't drink enough water and would get light-headed, and while she was nauseous, there was not a lot of vomiting because she was being treated with anti-sickness medication. By the time she reached 82, she had been disease-free for three years and her prognosis and quality of life looked good. But then she started getting pains in her lower back, and took a fall on the back steps of their house. We thought she'd hit her coccyx, so Anna went to the GP and had an X-ray. While they couldn't see anything, the pain continued, so she was put on Endone, a strong analgesia. I suggested she get a CT scan, which showed that the cancer had returned, and many of the nodes were pushing down on her back, which was the cause of the pain. I organised an appointment and arranged to be with her and her daughter Lety when she met with her oncologist, Professor Philip Beale.

'I could give you some more chemotherapy but you are three years older than last time,' Philip told Anna. 'You are not quite as well as you were then, but a lot of that could just be due to the pain. Because you had quite a good disease-free interval, we'll probably use the same drugs.' While there had been success with the previous regimen of drugs, there was no guarantee it would work a second time.

'I want to fight, Doctor,' she said, and I told her I'd help her every step of the way. We restarted chemotherapy and the first cycle reduced the nodes and nearly all her pain diminished.

That winter, when she was up to cycle five, I was on long-service leave and was away skiing when a snowboarder collected me on the Guthega Road and I flew up in the air and crashed down, breaking my L3 vertebrae on impact. I ended up in

Cooma Hospital for four long days. My brother Brian and his wife Joyce came to the rescue, picking me up from Cooma and taking me back to their place in Goulburn. Then a friend who I had been skiing with arranged to pick up my car from the snowfields and drive it back to Goulburn. She then picked me up from Brian and Joyce's and took me home to Sydney. I arrived on a Sunday afternoon, exhausted and in pain. The following Friday, my sister Loretta arrived from her home in Miranda to help me recuperate. She changed my bed and washed the sheets – she even did the gardening. That afternoon we went to visit Dante and Anna, but Anna was not particularly well. While Dante was showing my sister the new cupboards they'd bought for the spare room, Anna went to wash up the coffee cups and nearly collapsed at the sink. So I sang out to Ret because, with my broken back and only being out of hospital for seven days, I couldn't help. Helpless is not a state I like to be in.

Dante and Ret managed to get Anna onto her bed. After Anna had recovered enough to be safely left, Ret headed home and I also needed to lie down because I was still in pain and needed strong analgesia to deal with it. The next day, Anna got up early to go to the bathroom but collapsed again, this time in their hallway. For some reason Dante didn't come or call me, probably out of concern for my welfare. I only knew what had happened after Lety arrived at her regular time to take her father to the Saturday markets in Homebush.

'Mum's collapsed and I've called an ambulance,' she said when she came to my front door. With that, adrenaline kicked in and I immediately went next door. Anna was still conscious but had a pulse rate of about 180 and it was abnormal; I think she was in atrial fibrillation, which is when the heart's upper chambers or atria beat out of sync with the lower chambers or ventricles. She was also cold and clammy. The paramedics arrived quickly and I gave them her medical history, but she was deteriorating quite rapidly so they called for backup. When the other paramedic ambulance arrived, they managed to get a drip into Anna's arm, but she had no blood pressure and her pulse was still 180. She was rushed to RPA with Dante in the back of the ambulance.

Lety was cleaning up at her parents' house, but about 20 minutes after the ambulance had left she rushed over to my place again. 'The hospital has just called. I've got to get in there, they don't think Mum is going to make it.' While she dashed to RPA, I couldn't drive because of my broken back so I called on a friend who lived nearby to take me in. But, very sadly, by the time I got there, it was too late.

At RPA Emergency, there's a nice little room with soft lighting where they put the bodies of people who have passed away. We called in a priest and we all stood there around Anna's bed. She was given the last rites and we all said some prayers. She looked very peaceful.

Later, Dante and Lety told me they were asked earlier by hospital staff if they wanted Anna put on a respirator. They chose not to. In Anna's case, I feel this was the right thing to do. As a nurse, I can see that there comes a time when it's best to let go, and Anna was at that point. Later, I found out that her blood count was extremely low – her haemoglobin was 62, she had no white cells to fight off infection, her platelet count was 16 and her heart was racing. At the age of 83 and in the condition that she was, a choice needed to be made and the family did so after a discussion with the doctor. As a healthcare professional, it is my job to try to preserve and prolong life – that's part of our oath – but I knew that if Anna had been put on a respirator, she probably would have lived only a day or half a day longer. Would that have made any difference to her, or her family? We can't know for sure, and I do have the benefit of being able to look at it as a medical professional as well as from the perspective of a friend and neighbour of almost 30 years. But how do you differentiate between those two positions?

When my mother died, she had a massive stroke and we knew she wasn't going to survive. She waited long enough – two days – for her chickadees to come home, and that was her dying wish granted. I feel that God opened his arms to her then, and we would not have wanted it any other way. What it comes down to, for me, regardless of whether the person is my patient, my friend or my family member, is their quality of life. Was the right decision made in Anna's case? I believe the answer is yes. There were only about four or five hours between when Anna collapsed on the floor that morning and the time she passed away. That, I'd say, was a quick death. Dante found relief in that idea. He's always saying to me: 'I want to go the way my dear wife went.' Unfortunately, we usually do not have any choice in the matter.

Dante's been living in that same house for 58 years, has been my neighbour for three decades, and is now 89. He still takes out our rubbish bins and cooks me lunch when I'm home, and he would still like to mow my lawns – although it's a job I have since taken over.

As a healthcare professional and a long-term resident in my neighbourhood, I also know of a few other cases of cancer, and it just goes to show that no one is immune. There have been cases of lymphoma, uterine cancer, breast cancer and tonsil cancer among my friends and neighbours, and I am there for them when they need it. I'll go in to see them when they are getting treatment or advise them on what is likely to happen next. If there is a problem, I'm there to help sort it out.

Three weeks after I broke my back on the road from Blue Cow to Guthega and soon after Anna died, I was determined to continue with plans I had in place to travel to Italy as part of my long service leave to meet up with Sam Gibson, my Perth nurse practitioner colleague, in Rome. Many years earlier, I had heard of Sam's work as a clinical nurse consultant at St John of God Hospital, in Subiaco, and later met her at a cancer conference. She asked to have a look at the Sydney Cancer Centre, so I took her on a tour of Gloucester House where she was able to observe my role as a cancer nurse practitioner. It was soon after that visit that she decided she wanted to be a cancer nurse practitioner herself and would later complete an internship with me at Gloucester House as part of her course. Sam came to Sydney and stayed with me for two weeks and we both travelled to work at the Sydney Cancer Centre where she was able to see many of the clinical roles a cancer nurse practitioner plays in the treatment of a patient. We soon became great friends, and I was glad to spend time with her in Italy.

We were having coffee at the breakfast table in our hotel in Perugia when I received a surprise text from Gail O'Brien who knew of my impending retirement. She asked if I would accept the offer of a nursing scholarship under my name. I read the message with tears in my eyes and passed the phone over for Sam to read it too. *Of course*, I texted Gail, *it would be a privilege to accept such a wonderful offer and it would be such an honour.* That night Sam and I celebrated with prosecco. Chris O'Brien Lifehouse now raises funds for the Keith Cox Scholarship, which nurtures future clinical staff by offering financial support for nurses and allied health practitioners who wish to undertake further education.

If you're a nurse, people come to you with their ailments – and this continued even after my retirement. I've been a healthcare professional for almost 50 years, so I know how to feel a pulse or change dressings, advise someone on how to put on surgical stockings or what to say to Triple 0 or ambulance officers when a three-year-old neighbour swallows a 50-cent piece. There is a wide range of things that are now part of my make-up. You take an oath and that oath stays with you until you die, whether you need to help someone around the corner, on a plane or in a restaurant while you are supposed to be having a quiet dinner. You could hide away and not get involved, but whenever I could help anyone I would only be too willing to do so. You do what you have to do. I feel I was put on this earth to do a job, so I continue to do it where and when I can.

23

IS THERE A NURSE ON BOARD?

One somewhat dramatic example of helping wherever I could took place on a Qantas flight to Shanghai in 2014. Together with my colleague Kate White, a highly qualified nurse and professor of cancer nursing at Sydney University, I had been invited to speak at a cancer conference in Shanghai, to teach at Shanghai University School of Nursing and also to visit some cancer hospitals. There was also a side trip to the ancient water town of Zhouzhuang planned, where we would stay with locals and explore the city for a few days.

On the plane a couple of hours into the flight, I was coming back to my seat from the bathroom when I saw a woman in front of me holding a hot cup of tea in her hand. She seemed to be swaying and unsteady on her feet, so I took the cup out of her hand and put it on a nearby tray table. As I did so, the elderly lady lapsed into unconsciousness and fell into my arms, so I slowly lowered her to the floor. I was kneeling in the aisle, squeezed in between the seats by her side. I felt a pulse in her neck, but it was faint. A flight attendant soon came to help and I told her I was a nurse and explained what had happened.

'Look, I can't work on her here,' I said. 'We're going to have to carry her down to the bulkhead.' It was just past the toilet I had come from and there was more room there. The attendants were fantastic. 'What do you need?' they asked. 'Please get me a blood pressure machine and the emergency kit,' I replied.

Between us we carried the old woman up the aisle to the bulkhead where I took her blood pressure. It was something like 40 on nothing. That's bad. I could still only just feel the carotid pulse in her neck and it was very thready. By this time the chief flight attendant was hovering over us. 'My name's Mark. Are you OK?'

'I'm not quite sure what's going on with her,' I said, and explained a little about what was happening. He said, 'I'd better go and tell the captain because we might have to touch down somewhere.'

I asked the other flight attendants if the woman had anyone with her and I was told her husband was on board and they would locate him. The chief flight attendant then returned from the flight deck.

'The captain wants to be kept informed,' he said. 'If you want him to touch down, you need to tell him in the next 15 minutes because we'll be over Darwin.'

'OK,' I said. The patient, meanwhile, was semi-conscious but not alert and not responding. While there was more room in the bulkhead than in the aisle, it certainly wasn't ideal and I knew we needed to move the woman again if I was to treat her. I asked the flight attendants what our options were.

Then the captain came out, a really big fellow with a booming voice. He introduced himself – he was also called Mark – and I briefed him on what was going on. He offered to call the international medical team for flight emergencies in Atlanta, but I felt it was a little too early to make that decision, so we talked about other arrangements. Meanwhile, the passengers on the plane were craning their necks, trying to have a stickybeak to see what was going on.

The flight attendants, meanwhile, had been working on the problem of where we could move the woman. The plane was almost at capacity, but they had managed to commandeer one spare seat in a middle row in business class.

'If we can get her in there,' I said, 'I can treat her.'

With that, we carried her up the aisle and laid her flat on the base of the now reclined business-class seat. 'I think I'll move to give you a bit more room,' said the poor passenger in the adjacent seat. He'd probably paid a fortune for his ticket only to find himself down the back in cattle class.

'That'd be great,' I said. 'Thank you. Sorry.'

It was handy to have the seat next to the woman free so that I had room to work on her, and it also allowed me to have a look at what was in the medical kit. Fortunately, Qantas has very good medical kits, which included two 500-millilitre packs of Hartmann's, a plasma expander, which could at least help rehydrate this woman. I thought if I could get a drip in and rehydrate her, this would bring her blood pressure up. But I also suspected she had some sort of heart block and that was why her pulse was so slow. By this time there was a lot of other stuff happening. The husband, through an interpreter, said that the woman had fainted before and I asked if she had a heart problem.

211

'Yes. I'm not quite sure what it is but there was a similar event before,' he told one of the interpreting attendants.

Then Mark the flight attendant piped up. 'What do you want the captain to do? Do you want to touch down in Darwin?'

In the back of my mind I was thinking, *Do I have this plane land in Darwin, with a couple of hundred people on board, or do we keep on going?*

'Look, she's slightly better since we've got her here to the business-class seat,' I said. 'I think we'll be all right.'

While I could make decisions on her medical condition, the decision to land was not my call. Then the captain came back down from the bridge and told me, 'We've now overtaken Darwin, so if things don't improve, Jakarta's the next stop.'

'Right!' I said. 'OK.' That gave me a bit of time before I had to decide whether or not we needed to land in Jakarta.

Captain Mark went back to the cockpit and I addressed the cabin staff. 'If we can get a drip in, it would help.'

So I got everything ready until the only thing missing was the woman's consent.

'We're going to have to inform her of what I'm planning to do,' I said. 'I'm going to have to put this needle in her hand or her arm to give her the fluids. But I want her consent before I'm happy to do that.'

The woman was a little bit better at this stage and could respond to verbal commands. The interpreter explained to the woman and her husband what I wanted to do. Her response was clear.

'No,' she said, 'I'm not going to have it!'

'Well then, I'm not prepared to put it in,' I said to the crew. I wasn't in familiar territory, so didn't feel at all comfortable putting a cannula in without this woman's consent. After hearing this, Mark the flight attendant went back up to the flight deck to get the captain.

'What's the problem, Keith?' the captain asked.

I explained that we would have to stop in Jakarta because the woman's blood pressure was still 40 on nothing. Her pulse was about 38 and very thready, and while she had improved slightly, she was not taking any oral fluids and without a drip I simply couldn't get her all the way to Shanghai, which was still about eight hours away.

'Well, what do you want to do?' he asked.

'I want to put a drip, a cannula, in her arm, and give her these fluids.'

'Is that what she needs?'

'Yes.'

'Well, I'm the captain of this plane and what I say goes! So you tell her this is what's going to happen and that you'll be putting in the drip!'

The interpreter translated what the captain had said and the woman reluctantly agreed to the treatment.

'You'd better go and get my colleague Kate,' I told one of the attendants, 'because this woman is probably 80 years old and she's got very thready veins, and they're all shut down because she's dehydrated, so I'm going to need some help.'

A few minutes later, Kate arrived in business class and, after I quickly brought her up to speed, we examined the gear in the medical kit. While most of the equipment was very good, the cannulas were big – very big, like crowbars! Well, at least compared to the fine ones I was used to putting in for cancer treatment. So I was very glad to have Kate there to help me put it in.

I put the tourniquet on the woman's arm and started working through the veins on the top of her hand. She was elderly, dehydrated, with porcelain skin but no visible veins. So I started going, *Slap! Slap! Slap! Slap!* to try and bring the veins up. Nothing! Then I started working on her forearm: *Slap! Slap! SLAP! SLAP!* Nothing.

By this time, I'd been working on her for a full five minutes. So I closed my eyes and said a little prayer. 'Oh Lord, please can you help me put this cannula in?'

As I've mentioned, I used to be known as 'the King of Cannulation' or 'the Last Resort' when it came to putting cannulas into difficult-to-find veins. And while I had put thousands of cannulas in, and could probably do it blindfolded, I hadn't tested myself mid-flight, in a business-class seat, on an 80-year-old who couldn't speak English and was semi-conscious, lying flat out at 30,000 feet!

But then I opened my eyes and ever so slowly one little vein emerged. I pulled the skin taut, cannula in my fingers, thinking that there was no way this massive needle, a crowbar of a cannula, was going to fit into that tiny little vein. We were going to have to land in Jakarta! But, next thing I knew, it was in – even though it was like putting in a needle two sizes too big! So finally, the cannula was in, the Hartmann's was flowing and I held the IV bag aloft – almost victorious. But we weren't out of the woods yet.

'How are we going to do this, because I can't hold this IV all the way to Shanghai,' I said to Mark, the flight attendant. So he had a think and then disappeared for a moment, returning with a wire coathanger which he bent around to create a hook, then proceeded to hang the IV bag from the bulkhead. Problem solved, but that wasn't an end to all the excitement, either.

We were still a few hours out of Shanghai, with Kate checking in on me and the elderly passenger periodically, when Mark came back to business class. 'Keith, you won't believe this, but I want you to come and see a guy in Row 50. He's got a high temperature and he's not well.' So I headed back to economy with my Qantas medical kit, which contained the blood pressure machine and a thermometer.

I arrived to find a really big guy sitting with his partner. He can't have been very comfortable in the small economy seat, but that was the least of his worries. He didn't look well at all. I introduced myself and set about taking his temperature.

'Have you had any medical problems recently?' I asked.

'Oh yes,' he said. 'I went to the GP yesterday with a chest infection, and he put me on antibiotics.'

'Ah,' I said. 'OK. What were the antibiotics that you started on yesterday?'

'Oh no, I haven't started them yet.'

'Well, why not? What are you doing?'

And he said, 'I thought I'd just take them on the trip with me, just in case.'

I said, 'Well, now is your "*just in case*", as your temperature is 38.5°C!'

So his wife moved his beer out of the way and retrieved his antibiotics – amoxicillin, which is ideal for chest infections. I had a flight attendant get me some Panadol and instructed the passenger: 'Take these and don't drink any alcohol.'

By this time we were about 90 minutes out of Shanghai. This was not long after SARS, at a time when passengers with high temperatures were not being let off planes.

'If your temperature is not down in 20 minutes,' I told him, 'you won't be walking off this plane; you'll be carried off and you'll be going straight to hospital.'

I went back to my elderly patient in business class. By then she had eaten a little bit of soup and her signs were improving. The big guy, meanwhile, had literally just taken his medicine. So there we were, all buckled up for landing, me next to the elderly woman, my colleague Kate down the back, another sick patient in economy and several hundred other passengers on the flight, mostly unaware of all the drama that had unfolded between their take-off beers and morning breakfast buns and scrambled eggs.

After we hit the tarmac and the crew finally opened the doors, everyone else disembarked while the flight crew brought the hefty fellow and his wife up to business class to join me and the elderly woman. Soon after, a medical crew arrived on board. First, I briefed them about the elderly lady's condition, then I told the story of the passenger in Row 50 with the chest infection and the temperature of 38.5°C. They dealt with him first as his temperature was down and, luckily for him, they let him off the plane.

But I was not about to take the drip out of the elderly woman's arm because her blood pressure was still not that good, even though it had improved and her pulse was a bit stronger. She was on the second 500-millilitre bag of Hartmann's IV by this time, so the medical team got her ready to transport her to hospital. As we approached the exit with the elderly patient, her husband and all the medical team, we saw that waiting for us at the jet bridge, all lined up like a guard of honour, were Mark the captain, Mark the flight attendant and all the crew, who started clapping us off the plane as if we'd just finished a stage performance. After that, the elderly lady was taken off to hospital and I never heard another word about it.

The funny part is, years later, I was invited back to China to speak at a conference in Beijing. I flew up on a Friday, was flying back on a Sunday, and going back to work on Monday. This time I was treated to business class – not the new-style business class with the lie-flat beds, but the old one with the reclining seats. On the flight back from Beijing, about three or four o'clock in the morning, my back started aching, which it occasionally did since I'd broken it on my skiing holiday. I thought I'd get up and walk around and change from my Qantas pyjamas back into my clothes. So I was standing there holding my clothes when Maureen, the chief flight attendant, said, 'Mr Cox, do you just want to change your clothes?' And I said, 'Yes, please.'

'Just go into the captain's room there,' she said, pointing out a doorway to a room that contained a big chair, used by the flight crew to lie down for naps during the flight. 'I don't think he'll mind.'

So I changed out of my pyjamas into my clothes and came out with my PJs in my hand, and there, with his back to me, was a big tall guy in a captain's uniform peering into the toilets.

'Maureen, you need to get someone in there to mop up all that spilled water,' says a big booming voice.

'We're just about to do that, Mark,' she replied, adding, 'I hope you don't mind, but I let Mr Cox use your room to change.'

And with that, he turned around and with that familiar voice said, 'I know Keith,' and I said, 'I know Mark.'

It was the same captain from that eventful Shanghai flight.

'Oh, Keith,' he said. 'I could have done with your help on a flight a few weeks ago. This guy stood up to go to the toilet and promptly dropped dead!' Mark then told me they'd put an eye mask on the deceased, pulled a blanket up under his chin and sat him next to his wife until the plane hit the tarmac.

'Probably a little too late for that one!' I said.

24

NOT JUST PATIENTS, BUT PEOPLE TOO

There are not many people I don't like. I might say I find some people a bit weird, but I don't say I don't like them. Some just make a different impression than others. But as I've said, I treat everyone the same and try to maintain a positive outlook while I'm doing that, no matter what the patient's outcome may be.

Both Michael Boyer and Martin Tattersall liked me to get involved in the care of their patients for various reasons. Prior to Lifehouse, my office at Gloucester House 5 was so small that I could never see a patient in it, but I did have a little education room nearby that I could sit in, so patients could be brought in there to have a chat and to see if I could help.

As Michael often says, we'd also try to treat people as a team. Even when I became a cancer nurse practitioner and was able to order fluids or prescribe drugs or send patients for blood tests or ultrasounds or whatever, I did not work in isolation at Lifehouse. I worked as part of a group of other nurses and doctors and we were all part of the process. But I'd also share my mobile number with a patient and their relatives so they could ring me for advice or if they were having problems. While that isn't a common thing for nurses to do, I'd go the extra mile for a patient, just as I would for any friend. If you are in need, I'll be there for you.

BIAGGIO SIGNORELLI (1937–2008)

Biaggio Signorelli was a migrant who arrived in Australia from Sicily and worked with his family to build up a successful fruit and vegetable business in Lakemba, Willoughby and Blakehurst. But it was a second job in a factory making transformers that exposed him to asbestos, which inevitably cost him his life. Biaggio later expanded the fruit and vegetable business before diversifying into function centres in the 1970s and later built up the very successful Doltone House Group. In October 2007, as a direct result of exposure to that asbestos many years earlier, he was diagnosed with mesothelioma, an incurable form of cancer mainly on the wall of the chest. A patient of Michael Boyer, Biaggio was brought in by his son Paul to meet me at the then Sydney Cancer Centre. For some reason, even though we didn't have a lot in common, Biaggio liked me. And wherever Biaggio was, his son Paul was too. In 1990, at age 19, Paul had been involved in a serious truck accident and had almost died. During his recovery, Biaggio was always by his son's side. Now the roles had been reversed.

'You need to take me in to see Keith,' Biaggio would say to Paul, and the dutiful son would do his bidding. Dressed in pyjamas, dressing-gown and slippers, Biaggio would come into the outpatients' clinic with Paul. I'd ask what was wrong, assess his situation and sometimes if he was a bit dehydrated I'd give him some fluid, but half the time Paul reckoned his dad just wanted to come in to see me. Unfortunately, Biaggio didn't do well and was admitted to specialist palliative care at Calvary Hospital.

'Can you come and visit Dad? He wants to see you,' Paul asked me one day. So I went up to Calvary after work. Biaggio remained strong to the last and maintained a positive outlook that never waned, always believing that a hospital visit was just another hurdle that he would overcome. But he died on 30 May 2008, eight months after his initial diagnosis.

He had a big funeral at St Mary's Cathedral with 4000 people attending, including former prime ministers, former NSW premiers and Sydney's foremost business leaders. His was also the most amazing-looking coffin I'd ever seen. It was huge and heavy, so eight pallbearers were carrying it. The hearse had a police escort and the traffic had to be stopped as well to let the funeral cortege through. All the Doltone staff, in their black uniforms with the gold Doltone crest, lined the steps of St Mary's. This was a far cry from the life of the migrant who'd landed on the shores of Pyrmont in the 1950s with only a couple of suitcases and three kids in tow.

A bronze statue of Biaggio, his wife Phillipa and their seven grandchildren now sits on Wharf 12, Darling Island in Pyrmont and was unveiled in 2010 by then-Governor of NSW Marie Bashir. Named 'Life From A Suitcase', it is a tribute to all post-war migrants in Australia. I am now on the board of the Biaggio Signorelli Foundation, established by Paul and his two daughters, Anna and Nina, which creates awareness and helps those who have mesothelioma.

LUCINDA ANNE RETALLACK CAMPBELL (1991–2010)

Luci was a patient of Professor Martin Tattersall and was 17 when I met her. She was very sporty, played hockey, water polo, softball and netball and was a snowboarder. Luci was also very active in drama and painting. She had been diagnosed with a very rare sarcoma in her back. She was the only patient I'd ever come across with that type of sarcoma, and it's the only case I've ever seen since. Luci had surgery to remove the tumour, but the wound took a long time to heal. In addition, Luci had also accidently leant against a wall heater and seriously burnt her back and as a consequence, she was also a patient at Concord Hospital burns unit. Her back had to be dressed and cleaned once a day, which complicated the treatment and recovery from chemotherapy. I sought advice on the type of dressings she needed from nursing sisters who specialised in melanoma, as they were very experienced, and I began to dress Luci's wounds accordingly.

She then metastasised, which meant the cancer had spread and she needed chemotherapy. While it felt like years, it was only really a short time in which I got to know Luci, her family and all of her gorgeous schoolfriends who came to see her in Gloucester 5 while she was being treated. Luci celebrated her 18th birthday while at Gloucester 5 and even managed to get down to the Alfred Hotel for a legal drink with the nurses and a few friends, which highlighted her strength and desire to proceed with life. Luci's parents also used to ring me for advice and I'd go in specially to see her if she was in pain because I'd know what to do and how to manage it. Occasionally, while on Level 5, Luci would close a phone call by saying, 'I have to go now as my Nurse Practitioner has arrived.' Coincidentally, one great friend of Luci's was the granddaughter of Marie Bashir, then Governor of NSW. I'd known Marie from her work as a psychiatrist at Rivendell Adolescent Unit in Concord, and Marie would later present me with my OAM at Government House.

But Luci's chemotherapy treatment had a significant toll on her strength and health and sadly she headed down the palliative care path, which meant she was being looked after at home on Sydney's North Shore, until a stroke sent her to Royal North Shore Hospital and the palliative care unit at Greenwich Hospital a week later. Luci was amazing; she never really talked about death or dying but I'm sure that deep down she knew the truth of her situation. Her parents, Annie and Richard, and her brother, Edward, relied on my experience and friendship and would ask me to visit her when she was at Greenwich and I'd pop in when I could.

When I saw her, she was always wearing a pair of earphones and would often be engrossed in music, mostly oblivious to the visitors, just like during her time at RPA. I didn't ask what she was listening to but it helped her cope. Patients find all sorts of coping mechanisms that suit them while they are having treatment, or if treatment has failed and they know their time is short. I can picture her room on one of those occasions near the end: it had a window that overlooked the garden, it was night-time, and there was just a single lamp. Luci was lying on her bed, barely conscious. One of her aunts, Prue, was in the room with me. 'Keith, listen to this music with me,' she said, and we took an earphone each and listened to the song that had been playing on Luci's iPod. Prue and I looked at one another but didn't say a word; we just listened. It was the most beautiful song that I'd ever come across.

> *Stones taught me to fly*
> *Love taught me to lie*
> *And life taught me to die.*
> *So it's not hard to fall*
> *When you float like a cannonball.*

Luci deteriorated quite quickly and died later that night. She was 18. Maybe it was that particular moment, but Damien Rice's 'Cannonball' still brings tears to my eyes when I hear it. It has so much meaning and emotion connected to it for me – then and now. For Luci, it must have been her way to escape, her way of dealing with death and dying.

I was invited to her funeral in Canberra, an intimate one held at St John's Anglican Church, where her parents were married and where Luci had been christened. It was in January and on a stiflingly hot day. There was also another service at her Darlinghurst school, SCEGGS, which was attended by all the friends who'd visited Luci in hospital, as well as her teachers and four of us from the Sydney Cancer Centre. The Year 12 art prize at SCEGGS Darlinghurst now is named in her honour. While we all said our farewells to Luci that day, I remained in contact with her parents and went to their home a few times. I met up with her father Richard in Thredbo and we went skiing together down some of Luci's favourite runs. Within weeks of Luci's passing, her mother Annie also required treatment at Lifehouse, as secondary melanoma had returned. After a third diagnosis in 2013 and despite rounds of chemotherapy, radiotherapy and new, targeted trial therapies, Annie passed away in March 2015. Some families are beset by tragedy and it's often hard to fathom for those who are left behind.

ELLIOTT MILLER (1994–2016)

When Professor Martin Tattersall brought Elliott to see me, we connected straight away. Even though I only got to know him over a very short period – five months from diagnosis to death – he certainly made an impression on me and had a big impact on my life.

Elliott was a former St Aloysius College student who had enrolled at Sydney University and was doing quite well as an actor and director when he was diagnosed with sarcoma of his jaw. As with a lot of my patients, I told Elliott he could ring me anytime he needed. 'It's your favourite patient here, Elliott,' he'd say. After time in ICU, he had radiotherapy and chemotherapy, but none of that worked for him and the cancer spread.

Despite the rigours of his treatment, Elliott remained the most positive and likeable young man. As things progressed, though, I had difficulty controlling his pain, so I would call in the palliative care team to help. I was on holiday when Elliott was admitted to hospital for the last time and I received a call to say his mother was waiting for me to come in. Elliott was dying and didn't have long. He was hanging on for his girl-friend Bridget to return from a trip to the US and I was also told he was waiting for me to visit.

As soon as I arrived back at work, he was the first patient I went to see. In his room on Level 9 at Lifehouse, Elliott was unconscious. His mother Henrietta had stayed the night to be with him and when I entered, she was crying but was so pleased to see me. We both knew it would not be long.

I went up a couple of times to see him during my shift and then visited one last time before I left for the day. As I've said, the last sense to go is hearing, so I took his hand and said, 'Elliott, it's Keith here. You can let go now,' and he squeezed my hand very gently. Elliott died that night, 21 March 2016.

His funeral at Sydney's St Aloysius College was huge, and two Lifehouse staff and I went. We got there an hour early and by the time the service started, both the chapel and quadrangle were filled to capacity. It was as much a celebration of life as anything else. There were moving readings and heart-warming eulogies, and a couple of Elliott's mates offered some very funny stories and insights into his life. The crowd stood and applauded at the end. What an amazing young man who had so much to offer. It's a tragedy that we will never know what sort of life he could have led.

COOPER RICE-BRADING (1999–2017)

Cooper's cancer journey from diagnosis to death was also quite short, around 20 months, but what an impact he made on me and all those who came in contact with him.

Cooper was on a father–son trip to the Australian Open in Melbourne in late January 2016 when he complained to his father Colin of soreness in his arm. After being referred for a routine MRI, Cooper was told he had an aggressive and rare osteogenic sarcoma, or bone cancer.

When I first met Cooper, he was newly diagnosed. He was in Year 11 at Sydney Grammar School and was heading into his final year. He was also a talented rugby player, junior elite

AFL player, an avid Swans supporter and a representative crick-eter, with a right arm that was particularly skilful at taking wickets. Cooper was sent to me by Martin Tattersall because he knew I could provide the special attention this young man required.

Cooper and his parents came to my office in Lifehouse where we had a talk about his chemotherapy treatment, and I found him to be very intelligent from the start. We talked about fertility and, after his mother volunteered to leave the room to save him from embarrassment, his dad stayed for the remaining conversation in which we spoke about sperm banking. These sorts of subjects are often ones teenagers don't feel comfort-able talking about with their mum present – including what you have to do at the sperm bank or how many days it has been since you have had any sexual activity. And while it's not necessarily an intimate discussion, it's a delicate one, and a vital conversation that you need to have with a young patient who is about to undergo chemotherapy that could render them infer-tile for life. We also needed to talk about all the blood tests and other specimen tests, as well as the potential complications and side effects such as losing his hair.

In those first moments of our relationship, we got on extremely well. Cooper felt he could talk to me about anything and I always felt comfortable talking to him. At 17, body image is a huge thing and apart from a loss of hair, he'd already had part of his humerus removed from his left arm – not his bowling arm – and had a prosthetic bone inserted which had left a large scar. Overall, though, he was very accepting of how the changes were going to affect him.

Cooper started chemotherapy the week after we met. While he was never pessimistic, you can help keep a patient's spirits up by sitting down and listening, which I always tried to do. Cooper was a good example of the value in this, because he went through the surgery to remove part of his humerus, then had radiotherapy and had a disease-free interval for a little while. He even played cricket again and bowled, albeit without any hair, cheered on by his teammates, and he seemed determined to overcome any hurdle put in front of him.

But as often happens with these sarcomas, the cancer returned and Cooper relapsed. He needed to start a different type of chemotherapy treatment. His mother Tania later told the ABC that her son underwent 'a brutal regime of surgery, immunotherapy and chemotherapy, enduring ever-increasing pain' but added that the medical team at Chris O'Brien Lifehouse delivered 'the gold standard in treatment for osteosarcoma'.

Of all the patients I've treated, Cooper asked me some of the most intelligent but often the most difficult questions. 'Keith, why can't I have this as an outpatient?', 'Why do I have to come into the hospital?' or he'd say, 'I don't like the smell of the place', putting into words many of the feelings patients associate with chemotherapy. And he'd want all the details in my answers.

'We need to give you plenty of fluid before we start your treatment,' I'd explain. 'Then we need to alkalise your urine so that its PH level is not above 7, because if it is, this drug, which is excreted in the urine, will cause it to crystallise and can cause blockages. If that happens you could go into renal failure and then you'd have to go on dialysis. Then you need more fluid afterwards.'

'I understand all that,' he'd say. 'But why can't I drink all the fluid at home? Why can't I have the blood test that I had before? And I could be here at eight o'clock in the morning and have this treatment and the fluids and then I could go home at seven o'clock at night.'

So I sat down in my office and started working out a different regimen for Cooper, and then I went to see Martin.

'Prof, I've had a long discussion with Cooper. He doesn't like being in hospital. I'm trying to work out a better way but I need to treat him safely. I think his family are very responsible and they don't live very far away, so this is the regimen I've put together.'

'If you think it will work, I'm happy to give it a try,' responded Prof, and that's how Cooper had the next two treatments – as an outpatient. We put him in a single room, looking over Missenden Road up to Newtown, where he was treated before I sent him home with his oral fluids. If he hadn't questioned our existing methods, he would probably have continued his treatment in hospital. I've since heard that the existing treatment regimen is now changing, most likely because of him. I don't advocate for change just for the sake of change, but I did always try to show that if something is better, then we can change it. In a lot of the research that I conducted, I wanted to demonstrate that you could change practice, if you could see a better way and a safe way of doing it. Patients may not question you as a medical professional, but you can see they don't like being in hospital and they would prefer to be at home if their life expectancy is short.

In the last six to eight months before he died, Cooper kept questioning both Prof and me: 'Well, what new drugs are around for this treatment? What new research has been done? How long has this treatment been available for these people?'

'We've been using the same treatment for 40 years,' we'd tell him.

'Why aren't there new drugs?'

'Probably because sarcomas come in at about number eight on the top ten list of total number of cases of cancer.'

'Well, I appreciate that, but *I* have sarcoma.'

In the early hours, unable to sleep, he'd sit in his hospital bed at Lifehouse with his mother and they set about establishing a new sarcoma foundation to help with research and new treatments. He asked Professor Tattersall, his surgeon Richard Boyle, his radiation oncologist Angela Hong and myself if we would join the medical advisory board of this new foundation and, after a lot of hard work, the Cooper Rice-Brading Foundation was formed. Cooper pulled in many more favours and the foundation was launched at Doltone House in Sydney's CBD on 28 March 2017. Newsreader Peter Overton was MC but was running late as he was reading the 6 pm news bulletin, so radio host, family friend and Cooper's de facto big brother Michael 'Wippa' Wipfli stepped in until Peter arrived. Both personalities have been fully behind the foundation ever since. Cooper made a moving speech to those in the audience that night. It's on YouTube and still brings me to tears. How does a 17-year-old pull all that together, and get so many people on board?

Cooper died on 24 August 2017. His foundation has been up and running for four years now and we've gone from strength to strength. It focuses on raising awareness about sarcoma and raising money for research, as there wasn't much being done at all in that area, and it accounts for just 0.1 per cent of all cancer research. His parents and brother Mitchell are still the driving forces behind it, and they continue to raise funds and create awareness about osteogenic sarcoma, be it a banner at a Sydney Swans AFL match or a fundraising barbecue at the cricket.

MICHAEL WILLESEE (1942–2019)

Michael Willesee was one of Australia's most famous television journalists and presenters whose career spanned more than 50 years. But in Chris O'Brien Lifehouse, he was another cancer patient who needed my attention. I was introduced to him in mid-2017, the year of my retirement, by Michael Boyer, who had already been treating him for a few weeks. He telephoned me from his office upstairs to say that Michael Willesee was coming down and gave me a bit of background as to his condition. We used to see 1200 new patients a year at Lifehouse, and while we treated all patients the same way, the VIPs were often sent to me as I knew the ropes better than most. I had seen Michael Willesee at Lifehouse once or twice before our introduction, but I now knew he was fighting a losing battle with throat cancer. Sitting in my office, he was pleasant and spoke quietly and gently. We had a bit of a chat about his treatment but we were still waiting for some blood tests to come back and he also had to sign consent forms for a clinical trial, so we came to be talking about other things.

Michael was the son of WA Federal Labor Senator Don Willesee. He first made his name as a reporter on the ABC's *This Day Tonight* and *Four Corners* from 1967–1971. While he quickly earned a reputation as an interviewer and investigative journalist on the ABC, I remember him most from his days on *A Current Affair*, which started in 1971 on Kerry Packer's Channel 9. One of the most famous interviews he conducted much later was with Federal Liberal Party leader, John Hewson, in 1993. It was on a proposed goods and services tax, or the GST, and it became famously known as the 'birthday cake' interview. Many people think it was the interview that cost Hewson the chance of winning the 'unlosable election'. I'm not much into politics, although I have known quite a few politicians over the years, having gently twisted their arms for political donations for cancer causes.

Mike Willesee had already spoken of his cancer fight on the ABC's *Australian Story*, and also his return to the Catholic Church, so we talked briefly about the faith we shared. He said that after a long lapse, he had found 'comfort' in his return to Catholicism. But it was his WA connections that we spoke about most. Strangely enough, Michael's sister Colleen had joined the same order as my sister Fay, aka Sister Chrys: St John of God in WA. While they were not in the same intake, our sisters had both been there around the same period in the 1970s and knew each other quite well. Colleen had decided to leave the order after the reforms of Vatican II, but it was still quite the coincidence that our sisters had crossed paths and worked together all those years ago.

The job at hand now was to treat Michael, who had been prescribed a combination of targeted therapies. But he also had problems with side effects from the radiotherapy treatment, mostly with swallowing and a painful neck area from the radiation. Unlike chemotherapy, the side effects of radiotherapy can arise a lot further on into the treatment cycle and also linger for a long time afterwards. Michael had also been screened before I met him as he was on a clinical trial, and there are always a lot of hoops to jump through due to trial planning and logistics. So Michael had been coming in for a couple of weeks by the time I saw him.

There are four private rooms at each end of Level 1 of the day therapy unit at Lifehouse, and Michael wasn't feeling well from one of his treatments. That was the first day I met Colleen. Her brother introduced us; he had already told his sister of our mutual connection. From that day on, whenever Mike came in, Colleen was with him. I got to like them both very much over that short amount of time. While Michael had faced some personal and professional challenges in his life, as we all do, when I met him, he was a very nice, personable and gentle man. On 1 March 2019, at the age of 76, Michael Willesee AO and TV Hall of Fame member died of throat cancer.

CAITLIN DELANEY (SURVIVOR)

Caitlin Delaney was and still is an amazing person. The young mother of two had been diagnosed with Stage 4 ovarian cancer in 2017 when she was 39, and I was called in to see her at Lifehouse as they were having trouble getting a needle in and she had a panic attack during her second chemo treatment. As I've mentioned, I was known around the building as the King of Cannulation so I was called in to make another attempt to insert the cannula and help alleviate her anxiety.

'The more they try, the worse it is and I'm getting very stressed,' she said as she sat there with her husband Kevin.

'I'd like to try something different,' I said. I've been taught many techniques to get needles in arms over the years and while some call this method 'imagining' or relaxation therapy, it's a technique known by many names. It had worked on some other patients before, but not all, so I told Caitlin to close her eyes and asked her to describe a place where she felt safe and a place where she had enjoyed a good time. She did as I asked and started to describe to me a scene of a beach spread out before her at Huskisson on the NSW south coast.

'What does the beach look like?' I asked.

'The waves are coming in on the sand and it's beautiful and white.'

'What colour are the waves?'

'They have white peaks on them but the water is this most beautiful blue colour.'

'Is the sun shining?'

'The sun is beautiful. It's shining on the water, but it's also shining on us and I feel nice and warm.'

'What else is happening?'

'Kevin has just arrived.'

'What's Kevin got?'

'You know what he's brought?'

'No, what has he brought?'

'He's brought my favourite champagne.'

'Which is your favourite champagne?'

'Billecart-Salmon.'

'That's funny, that's my favourite as well!'

I had another nurse with me because it's hard to take a patient through this process while also trying to put a cannula in their arm. But never at any stage did I mention to Caitlin that she might feel a little scratch or prick. She was sitting in one of the nice pod chairs we have at Lifehouse, her eyes closed. The needle was in and Kevin was watching as the drip started to flow.

'Caitlin, you can finish this beautiful story if you'd like to, but the chemotherapy is up and running.' And with that, she opened her eyes.

'That's a miracle,' she said, 'I didn't feel a thing.'

That was the start of our beautiful friendship.

Although Caitlin is still fighting cancer, she and Kevin have bought their first home which they've renovated. While Caitlin had various procedures and treatments such as immuno-therapy and radiotherapy she has had no further operations since I retired. Despite all this she's very proactive and set up a GoFundMe page, which raised enough money for the next year of her treatment. Caitlin has also established CareFully, a foundation which aims to equip healthcare professionals with the tools and training to provide compassionate, patient-centred care. She also advocates and raises money not only for the Australia New Zealand Gynaecological Oncology Group's Save the Box campaign but for Ovarian Cancer Australia and Rare Cancers Australia as well.

Patients are all different, of course. They would often talk to me of their fears for the future, their concerns about treatment and its side effects, such as losing their hair, or the impact treatment would have on their relationships, their families, their finances. They would even raise their fears about death. It's one of the things I miss most since retiring – the people. Whether famous or not, patients usually want someone who will listen. Their mind, body and soul are what I treat – the whole person, not just the illness. You make the time to talk to them and it might be only a couple of minutes, but they could be crucial minutes. I'd often get the feeling that something else was going on, and while I'd focus on the symptoms, I'd realise there was some-thing they needed to talk about. I'm happy to listen, to give you some advice, but there are others better trained in some areas. That's one good thing about working within a team: all these people can work comprehensively on a plan to treat the one patient as a whole. I'm now very experienced in having those discussions, but I also know when it would be better for them to speak to a counsellor, a psychologist, an exercise physiologist, a social worker or a dietician. You can't be an expert in all areas, but I can recognise when those referrals are needed, and help patients make an appointment with the right person.

This is part of what Chris O'Brien was trying to achieve before he died: a comprehensive cancer centre that had everything in one place to assist patients and enable them to have holistic care. A patient didn't have to go here, there or somewhere else to get that advice or treatment. When Chris O'Brien Lifehouse opened in 2013, it was a beautiful, modern building without the atmosphere of a hospital. It was open and bright and there was a real sense of welcoming. A piano or harp could be playing in the foyer where you were greeted by a receptionist before you headed up to your single rooms, with an en suite bathroom and possibly a balcony with views of the city. It was those ideas, that warm feeling, that philosophy in one safe space that is now part of Chris O'Brien's legacy, all there in the standalone cancer centre that is Lifehouse.

25

A SHARP MIND DULLED
BY DEMENTIA

MARTIN TATTERSALL (1941–2020)

When Martin Tattersall set up a role for me at RPA when I returned from England, it would be the beginning of a 43-year working relationship. He was a hugely important mentor and educator for me, and also a great researcher. He was always questioning me about why we were doing something in a particular way, and his inquisitive nature rubbed off on me. For instance, I'd ask, 'Can we give this person their treatment as an outpatient instead?' or 'Why don't we try a different method?' Martin was also the author of several hundred medical research papers, and, along with Dr Derek Raghavan, was one of the first people to prompt me to put my own expertise down in writing. Martin not only educated nurses, he also educated doctors and allied health workers. He taught in developing countries such as Afghanistan when the war was on, and in Pakistan and Papua New Guinea, sharing his knowledge and encouraging me to do the same. His philosophy was: if you know you can do something to help in developing or underdeveloped countries, that's what you should do.

Not only was Martin a good mentor and teacher, he was also a good friend. In those early days, I was not just part of the team, I was *in charge* of the team, and had to lead from the front. Often, as a nurse, it's not easy to be dealing with patients and their relatives at the same time as handling staffing issues, let alone the different personalities across the board. But Martin was always there. If I went to him to talk, he would always listen. Moreover, on more than one occasion, if he recognised that the morale of the unit might be a bit low, he'd say: 'Keith, let's organise something. How about we all have lunch at my place?' So he would invite up to 100 medical, nursing and other staff over to his waterside house in Woolwich. He and his wife Sue would open their beautiful home to all of us, and all Martin's 'toys' were there for us to play with – a boat and windsurfers among them. He'd done well and was willing to share that success with the staff.

In July 2017, I was 68 and still working 11–12 hours a day. I'd already had the skiing accident which broke my back, and that was on top of another health issue: atrial fibrillation (AF), which is when the electrical impulse of the heart misfires. It had been first diagnosed in 2011 after I had finished a regular morning gym session and felt a little shortness of breath after walking home. At work later that day I met Martin Tattersall, and as we climbed a flight of stairs together I felt short of breath again. After feeling a further flutter around my heart, an ECG was taken by one of my nursing colleagues which indicated I was in AF, which I refused to believe. We consulted my cardiologist colleague David Celermajer and he confirmed the diagnosis. The following morning I had an ECO which showed I also had a slightly leaky mitral valve. I had to be cardioverted, a procedure conducted under general anaesthetic where the heart is stopped then restarted to get it back into sinus rhythm. I've had to be cardioverted a couple of times since. With those health issues in mind, and after taking some of my remaining annual and long service leave, I was scheduled to retire in November that year. I loved my work; I loved doing what I did, but if I were to finish, I wanted to finish on top. Decision made.

To mark my retirement, Sue and Martin Tattersall held a wonderful cocktail party for me at their Woolwich home, and people gathered from all over, from medical professionals and colleagues to mutual friends. Professor Dick Fox and his wife, Julie, even flew in from Melbourne for the occasion. Dick was one of the three top cancer doctors in NSW who had helped establish modern-day cancer care at RPA. The oncology triumvirate included Dick, Martin and Dr Bob Woods – later a federal senator – all of whom had given me references when I left BP4 to go to England all those decades ago.

At work, just prior to the party (one of three leaving functions held for me), I noticed that Martin was starting to be a bit forgetful. Fellow colleagues and friends had also started to recognise that Prof wasn't quite himself. As I was still on painkillers for my broken back, I thought it might just have been my imagination, but all our mutual fears about Martin would soon be confirmed.

About a year after my retirement, on the wharf at Woolloomooloo, on the edge of Sydney Harbour, a big dinner was held for Prof to celebrate 40 years of his work in cancer medicine in

Australia, with 100 guests invited to help. Professor Alan Coates, a longstanding oncologist and friend of Martin, gave a lovely tribute, and Martin's eldest son Stephen spoke about his father's awards and achievements. Afterwards, Martin stood to respond and began his speech. He opened his mouth but was only able to utter a few words before he stopped in his tracks, unable to pick up his train of thought. The room was silent. I felt for him. Everybody did. All those at the dinner knew immediately that this was going to be some sort of farewell, but we were determined to focus on the positive aspects of his career.

The following morning at Lifehouse a research day was scheduled to be held in Martin's honour, and medical colleagues and nursing staff gathered to hear about the depth of research he had conducted over four decades of practice. As part of this I gave a presentation about his involvement in nursing, telling the audience how Prof had an unwavering dedication to patients and their families, always putting them first. He was always available to talk, contactable at any hour of the day or night. I told them how I remembered attending social events with him, suddenly noting his absence and finding him off to one side, answering a call from a patient or a member of their family. This was to say nothing of his kindness, generosity and sense of humour. Everyone liked Prof. The achievements of his lifetime were simply innumerable.

In 1977, aged just 36, this young cancer expert from the UK was appointed Professor of Cancer Medicine at the University of Sydney, and later that same year founded the Royal Prince Alfred Hospital Department of Medical Oncology. Later, he became the longest-serving professor in the Sydney University medical faculty. He is now considered one of the 'fathers' of medical oncology in Australia. He was a skilled educator, deeply committed to teaching the next generation of medical oncologists, who found his lessons highly engaging and always delivered with humour. Many of Martin's students have gone on to head other cancer centres and research institutes across Australia and the world. Martin also travelled widely to developing countries, helping to educate healthcare professionals about cancer and oncology. He was one of the first to understand the importance of communication and psychological research in cancer care. He was a member of the World Health Organization Cancer Committee and a Life Member of the International Union Against Cancer Roll of Honour. He amassed numerous awards, not least of which was the Medical Oncology Group of Australia Cancer Achievement Award in 2000. In 2003 he was made an Officer of the Order of Australia for services to medicine, and he also chaired the Australian Drug Evaluation Committee from 1997–2008.

I did not see Martin and Sue much after those gatherings as I was winding down at Lifehouse and RPA myself, but Martin's decline progressed quickly. In early 2019, I saw him standing on the side of the road near my home in Drummoyne and he was carrying a pair of brogues. He looked lost. 'Hi, Prof,' I said, and he looked at me as if I was a stranger. 'Have you just picked up your shoes from the bootmaker? Are you going to your car?' I asked, and he continued to look at me blankly. 'Yes,' he said eventually, so I waited until he crossed the road because I thought he was going to get knocked over. I later found out that his wife Sue had sent him off to pick up the brogues from the shoe repairer and had agreed to wait for him at a bakery down the road. But after he had picked up his shoes, he had forgotten where he was, and Sue had no idea where he had gone. In hindsight, I should have known something was badly wrong.

In August 2020, I received a call from Sue.

'If you'd like to visit Martin, I suggest you come sooner rather than later,' she said.

As soon as I was able, I hurried over to their home. Martin had been discharged from North Shore Private Hospital a fortnight beforehand, returning home to spend the last of his days with his family. I arrived at their house and Sue invited me into the kitchen for a cup of tea. As two medical professionals, we talked matter-of-factly about the treatment Martin was receiving.

'It's hard,' I said, 'and you must be exhausted.'

It was a good opportunity for Sue to talk through the process and while we sat drinking our tea, I just listened. She'd hardly been getting any sleep. In the early stages of Martin's return home, she'd have to get up in the middle of the night to take him to the bathroom. But as his condition declined, they set Martin up in a bed in the living room, inserted a catheter, and put him on morphine and the sedative midazolam, which was part of his palliative care.

The huge living room featured a big fireplace down one end and several French doors leading to an open verandah over-looking the Lane Cove River with views across Woodford Bay. Martin had carers, nurses and other assorted medical staff hovering around him 24 hours a day. They had rearranged the room so there was plenty of space for the carers as well as medical equipment and they had music playing – Mozart, Bach and Vivaldi – not too loud, but audible in the background. It was such a picturesque outlook, but when I turned to look at Martin, I was shocked and he appeared very distressed. I have seen many people in the late stages of their lives and, while I didn't say it out loud, I knew Prof was not going to last long. Any patient's quality of life at this late stage is not good, so the aim is to keep them as comfortable and pain-free as possible and alleviate any anxiety they may have. I moved towards him and put my hand near his. He took it and squeezed it lightly. A palliative care nurse had been giving him his medication, so he was in a daze, and as he was bed-bound, he needed to be turned regularly, so the nurse in me moved him onto his side. When I touched him, he was just skin and bone. I thought he'd probably pass away in the next few days, so I told Sue I'd come over again later.

'Don't leave it too long,' she said as we went back into the kitchen. As much as she meant this for Martin, I also think she liked having company.

'Just before you go, I want to ask you something,' Sue said. 'Will you do part of the eulogy at his funeral?'

She was getting very teary and I was as well and we hugged. Martin had taught me so much, and we had worked so well together over our two lifetimes of medical care. We'd shared so many patients and he'd entrusted so much to me. He gave me so many opportunities as a nurse and a researcher, and he always valued my opinion and my input. The answer was never in doubt.

'I'm honoured to do it but I might get a bit upset,' I told Sue. 'I'm a bit of a sook.'

'That's OK,' she said. 'It will be from the heart. I don't want people talking about all his achievements. I want you to talk about him as a person.'

At his death, aged 79, Martin had published more than 600 medical papers; he had been awarded more than $20 million in research grants, supervised more than 20 PhD and MD research students, and had his work recognised with an Order of Australia. But to me, he was a great friend and an even greater mentor. For a man with such a renowned medical brain to be brought low by dementia, stripped as he was of the capacity to think rationally and to reason and to control his own body, is difficult to fathom. After all those years dedicated to helping others, travelling the globe and educating people, to end up standing on the road, clutching a pair of brogues and wondering where on earth he was, is such an unfair end to an extraordinary life.

26

CARING FOR MY OWN FAMILY

I am still very close to my family and we keep in regular contact. As we grow older and while COVID-19 has kept us apart physically, we are often on the phone, getting updates via calls or texts. Sadly, my eldest sister Fay, aka Sister Chrys, has dementia. After moving back to Goulburn to nurse at the hospital and care for Mum and Dad, Fay stayed for a few years before moving to Melbourne to work, then returned to WA to retire soon after her 70th birthday in 2005. Still living in Perth, Fay is now cared for by nuns from her own St John of God order – the same order who looked after my mother before she died. Before COVID-19, I'd head over once or twice a year or for significant life events, like Fay's 80th birthday.

When my other sister Coral retired from nursing many years ago, she and her husband Owen moved from Karratha to Perth. After living in a large house in Cloverdale, they decided to downsize to a three-bedroom villa in Kewdale, within easy distance of just about everything they needed – and only 20 minutes away from Fay. When I'd fly over, I'd always stay with Codge, but when COVID-19 prevented me from going, she kept me up to date on Fay's condition. Fay has been pretty much bed-bound for a decade now, but on her last birthday, her 86th, Coral, now 84, went to visit and Fay was sitting upright, moving her hand up and down in time with the music they were playing to her.

A few years after Coral and Owen moved to Perth, Owen was diagnosed with colorectal cancer and during surgery doctors discovered the cancer had spread to his peritoneum. They did manage to come to Sydney for Christmas that year, but returned home to Perth soon after where they found the cancer had progressed to Owen's liver. The prognosis was not good. Coral and I spoke on the phone often during that difficult period, and as I had a lot of leave up my sleeve, I said I'd go over to help. Like many cancer patients, Owen wished to die at home. With my cancer background and Coral's expertise as a nurse, we could make that happen, so I booked a flight. But on the weekend before I was due to leave, home care became too difficult for the palliative team at Owen and Coral's home, and Owen was admitted to Hollywood Private Hospital. Sadly, Owen died the day before I was due to fly out. I went anyway and was able to help Coral organise what needed to be done. Coral is practical, although maybe that's not the right word; she wouldn't have liked to see Owen suffer any longer but still misses him greatly. You can never fully prepare for the death of a loved one, but their family had time enough to prepare for what was to come, which was some relief.

My sister Dawn was born two years after Coral. She went to work in an electrical store in Goulburn straight after finishing school but didn't stay long as she decided she wanted to join the Air Force. She started her training in Mount Cook in Victoria and then transferred to Stockton near Newcastle. There she met her husband, Leo, who was a paratrooper in the army and used to come across to Stockton to do his jumps. They have a son, Steven, and a daughter, Vicki, who is now one of three in the next generation of our family to have become a nurse. Vicki works at Grafton Base Hospital, not far from her mum, Dawn, who is now aged 83 and lives in a nursing home nearby. My grandniece Ashley, granddaughter of Coral, also wants to become a nurse and is currently in training in Perth. Corinne, another of Coral's granddaughters, is also completing her general nursing course.

My brothers Brian, now 81, and Ronnie, 79, were always quite close when they were young. They both loved cars – Brian was a Holden man while Ronnie favoured Fords – and used to wash and polish their cars early every Saturday morning before heading to Goulburn, where they'd cruise up and down Auburn Street. Goulburn was also where they went for entertainment – and to meet prospective partners, which was how Brian met Joyce, who came from a big property out at Bannister, up Crookwell way. My older brothers were country boys; they liked the land and that sort of life. Brian started shearing and Ronnie worked on a local farm for the Sullivan family. The Sullivans had the first television in Cullerin, so we used to head to their house to watch their TV in flickering black and white. Ronnie later worked in soil conservation until he retired, and until recently he still worked for a farming family on the weekends. Brian stopped shearing sheep and fencing work when he was 80. Ronnie's wife Susan survived breast cancer 18 years ago, so I was there for that and was able to help her through it. Sadly, after all that, she has now been diagnosed with lung cancer and it has spread to the brain.

Judy, now 76, is next in line. She survived the 2003 Canberra bushfires which killed four people and destroyed 500 houses around her but left her own home intact. She and her husband Nick stayed to repair the heat and smoke damage to the house, but soon sold up and moved to Perth. Nick recently died after being diagnosed with throat cancer.

I am after Judy, and Loretta and Vincent came after me. Loretta is now grandmother to five granddaughters and she dotes on them all. Not long after finishing school, Vincent caught the nursing bug too and came to Sydney to start three years of psychiatric nursing training at Broughton Hall in Callan Park. He then applied to do his general nursing training, but didn't want to come to RPA because I was already there! While we three youngest ones – Ret, Vincent and me – were always close, Vincent coming to work with me at RPA would have been a bit crowded, I suppose. So off he went to Prince of Wales Hospital instead, where he completed two years general training. Now 66, Vincent is on the verge of retirement from St Vincent's Private Hospital in Darlinghurst after more than 35 years of service. I am glad that after commuting for three hours every day, he now gets to enjoy his Blue Mountains garden.

I feel blessed to be growing older with so much family still around, and to see a new generation go into nursing. I think Bill and Pansy would have been proud too.

27

SIX DEGREES

You've probably heard of the idea of six degrees of separation: that all people are six or fewer social connections away from each other. As I have done the rounds, literally, I have met quite a few people in the course of my life. So it is not uncommon for my name to crop up or for it to be recognised. 'I know Keith Cox!' Or as someone joked, 'I know someone who knows Keith Cox!' For me, it's a pleasure to be able to introduce a friend or a contact of mine to someone who may be able to help somebody else in need. I guess that's how it goes.

Unbeknown to me, I was nominated for an Order of Australia Medal, and found out via a letter sent to me from Governor-General Michael Jeffery in Canberra, on behalf of Her Majesty, Queen Elizabeth II. The letter, dated 10 April 2007, was headed 'Honours-In-Confidence' and asked if I would accept a citation in the Queen's Birthday Honours List: *For service to nursing, particularly in the field of oncology, and to the community through a range of youth, church and welfare organisations.* I felt very honoured and a little excited but had to keep it top secret until just before the announcement on the Queen's Birthday weekend in June of that year.

On the day of the investiture ceremony, held in September, I was allowed to bring three people as guests. So I invited Ret, her husband Tony and their son Luke, who is also my godson and a police inspector. The investiture was at Government House in Sydney, and as my citation was read out, I was standing in the doorway of the French doors leading from the verandah when the Governor of NSW, Marie Bashir, looked straight at me. As mentioned, we had known each other at RPA, and she had worked in adolescent psychiatry. She took my hand as she lifted the golden OAM. 'How lovely one of our nurses has been recognised,' she said as she attached the award to my lapel. Later, as we celebrated with champagne and a morning tea in the garden, Marie and I talked about my award and how lovely the day was, and we had a snap taken in the garden. Her husband, Nick Shehadie, came over. 'Marie, when Keith received his award I thought you were going to cry.'

'Well, I nearly did,' she said.

After receiving my OAM, I became a life member of the Order of Australia Association. In 2019, the association organised a Battlefields Tour of Europe. I was a bit nervous as I hadn't travelled by myself before and I didn't know anyone else on the tour. We had drinks and dinner on the first night, overlooking the Bosphorus in Istanbul. While I was chatting with one group, a woman arrived in a wheelchair. This was Dawn Ferguson, a former nurse who received her OAM in 1998 for her service to the GFS (originally Girls' Friendly Society), an Anglican

Ministry, and her work with the Linnet Choir of Sydney. We started chatting and I told Dawn that I was also a nurse. Coincidentally, both of us had trained at Royal Prince Alfred, but decades apart. I told her I had trained under a matron by the name of Margaret Nelson and Dawn revealed that they had been nursing students together, back in the day. Dawn was accompanied on the trip by her two adult sons, Lindsay and Rick.

During those three weeks together, on our tour of Turkey and the Western Front, I got to know everyone in our small group. While we all had something in common, the Fergusons and I spent a bit more time together and it was then that Rick told me his eldest son, Daniel, had Limb Girdle Muscular Dystrophy Type R1 (formerly known as 2A), a rare disease characterised by progressive weakness of the limbs and girdle muscles, especially those around the hips and shoulders. Later, in Paris, on the last day of our trip, I met Rick's other son Aaron. I was later invited to Rick's birthday dinner at a restaurant in Leichhardt where I would meet his other children, including Daniel.

While they had told me a little about Daniel's muscular dystrophy, none of it made much sense to me, let alone Limb Girdle Type R1. I could see that Daniel was headstrong and independent, but the simple daily tasks we all take for granted were becoming increasingly difficult for him to manage by himself, and as much as he wanted to do everything, those around him would have to step in at some stage. Daniel is now in his late 30s, lives independently, has a jewellery business and still drives a car. He also has a battery-operated mobile chair which helps if he needs to walk long distances. But in a few years, he will likely be in a wheelchair and his parents will need help looking after him as they get older.

After we returned home, I invited Rick and his wife Therese, also a nurse, to take a tour of my own personal battlefield, Lifehouse. We share the same faith and when they come over to Drummoyne on Sundays, we all attend Mass at St Mark's church.

'There's a reason why we have become good friends,' I said one Sunday after church as we headed down the street for a coffee. 'But I'm not quite sure why the Lord has brought us together.'

'It will all be revealed one day,' Rick said.

'Well, I don't want to get "up there" before I find out,' I said pointing skyward.

My inquisitive nature got the better of me and I started to seek out information on LGMD R1, but the more I drilled down, the more confusing it became. Over those first six months, we built up a great bond, and with some of my motivation and medical experience and the determination of Daniel's parents, we had agreed that we must do something that will not only assist Daniel but other sufferers of this disorder as well. So we set up a board, and the Daniel Ferguson Foundation was formed, with me as a medical advisor. The foundation now aims to raise awareness, advance more specific medical research into the condition, and improve the quality of life for those living with it.

Before we even thought of the idea for a foundation, and through our new friendship, Daniel made a beautiful white gold ring for me which features a sign of the cross. I also met Rick's youngest daughter Elyse and we talked about the ring. Elyse was engaged and showed me the beautiful ring which Daniel had made for her. It was stunning.

'I don't suppose you know any priests?' she asked.

'Well, as a matter of fact, I know quite a few,' I said. Elyse explained that she wanted a younger priest, someone to whom she and her fiancé Kieran could relate. I just happen to have a neighbour, Luke Meagher, whose brother Matthew was recently ordained. Like me, Luke is one of nine children, and his father is a colorectal surgeon at St Vincent's Hospital while his mother is a physician. I had a lunch at my place to introduce everyone to each other. Over the course of our lunch, Matthew agreed to officiate at Elyse and Kieran's wedding and he was thrilled at the thought of helping his first couple to tie the knot.

After several COVID delays they did eventually get married, but without Matthew officiating. Although if anyone else wants to get married by a nice young priest, I know someone who fits the bill.

One of the reasons six degrees of separation happens so often in my life is that I have always valued being an active part of the community, whether that's at the hospital or on my street. After my return from the UK, I felt the need to do more for the poor, so I thought of joining the local St Vincent de Paul group and considered becoming an acolyte, helping out at church services and giving communion. But they were just thoughts until I moved to Drummoyne, after which everything happened quite quickly. Soon after I moved, we parishioners at my church, St Mark's, were addressed by a St Vincent de Paul volunteer one Sunday night at six o'clock Mass. We were told of a recruitment drive as there were only four volunteers left in the group, and all of them were elderly. So eight of us joined that night. Peter Burbidge was then president and had great leadership and vision. Not long after we started, he asked if I was prepared to take on the role of treasurer. I'm not bad at maths, having spent all that time in our shop in Cullerin, and it wasn't quite as complicated then as it is today. I agreed and we got to work.

About a year later we got a letter from Father John Conway saying St Canice's Kitchen in Potts Point needed parishes to organise volunteers who could come on a Sunday and provide a meal for the less fortunate. The subject was raised at the St Vinnies meeting, and we all agreed we'd do it. One of the volunteers was Terry Boccalatte, a longstanding St Mark's parishioner, so I took on coordinating one group and Terry took on another. We provided tablecloths and table service, delivering meals to the tables of the Roslyn Street dining room. I'm still good friends with some of the group, including Michael Harrington who joined the same night as me. The president Peter Burbidge was quite old even then and had a carotid embolism and needed surgery, so he stepped down from the presidency and asked me if I would take on the overall coordination of the kitchen. Like everything else I am usually asked to do, I said yes. I've now been with our local Vinnies for almost 30 years and, before COVID hit, I'd been serving Sunday meals at Canice's Kitchen for almost as long.

Back then, I also told our local priest, Father John, that I'd like to become an acolyte, so I enrolled in a six-week course, one night a week at St Fiacre's at Leichhardt. After completing the course, I was installed as an acolyte by Bishop Geoffrey Robinson by a ceremonial tap on the shoulder. It was then that I reconnected with Father Vince Redden, who I had known briefly when he was a chaplain at RPA. He also knew my friend Father Bob quite well, as Father Vince was a major influence on Bob getting into St Paul's Seminary. So I was already an acolyte at St Mark's, helping to serve at Mass, by the time Father Vince was posted there. Father Vince is an old-school parish priest, I was a nurse and we both had a great connection to Royal Prince Alfred, so it wasn't long before we became good friends. We would talk about how to help people who were dying or who were having difficulty with their impending death, and the pain and suffering that they were enduring. He used to help guide me through it. He is in his 80s now and we stay in contact. I constantly tell him how much he increased my faith and how much stronger I am for him being there.

People say to me, 'How can you be always giving? You serve the poor, you do this and that, you've been looking after sick people all your life.' But I think I am rewarded ninefold. I have people there, too, if I need them. My faith and my passion have brought these people into my life, and not only made me a better person for having known them but also by giving me people with whom I can share and cherish the ups and downs. I have been very fortunate not to have had many downs.

These days I have cardiomyopathy and on occasion will go into atrial fibrillation which causes my heartbeat to become irregular and sends me back into the hospital every once in a while, but I never ask God, 'Why?'. It's hereditary, and everyone gets sick at some stage. It's what we do with the time that we have that is important. Recently I am getting a little bit more sensible about my 'retirement' and not taking on too much because I don't want to end up back in hospital. But that doesn't stop me from organising our annual street party, which has been going for the last 26 years, even during COVID-19. At one stage we had 150 people turn up and we had games and rides and the council even had to block off the street.

Also, I try my best to be nice, polite and friendly. I think, judging by the responses I get from people – like my neighbours dropping off a freezer full of food when I am sick, or people asking if they can do anything for me, or stopping in with a takeaway coffee for me – that the feeling is well and truly reciprocated. Tania Rice-Brading, mother of my former patient Cooper, came and picked me up to take me to an appointment one day, and she had made four different meals for me. I can see all the love that people are showing me, and I am so grateful. Even when I am sick, I rarely sit down to watch a movie or do nothing. I think it's a waste of time when there is so much to do out in the world. During COVID-19, for instance, I was called back to work at Lifehouse and asked if I could consult with patients via Telehealth from my house. I headed back into Lifehouse, undertook training in COVID-19, and once that was done, they brought all this computer gear to my place to set it up in my home office. I was glad to help.

This I know for sure: if we all tried to do something good for our fellow man or woman, the world would be a lovely place.

28

NO LONGER A DEATH SENTENCE

When I started in nursing in the 1970s, being told you had cancer was pretty much considered the kiss of death – no matter your age. By the 1990s things had improved, but we still didn't have a cancer ward at RPA and patients were scattered throughout the hospital, lying in a bed, or sitting in a chair in the Brown Street outpatients' department with a cannula in their arm, hooked up to a drip. Women being treated for breast cancer, for example, would come into the outpatients' department and have their treatment over several hours or even several days. We used to enter their names into a big admission book and I'd have three to four admissions a day scheduled for chemotherapy, but by 4 pm, the hospital still wouldn't have beds available so a patient would just be sitting there waiting as their particular treatment required a bed or chair.

Over time, little by little, things improved. But throughout all those years, people such as Michael Boyer and I were always looking for new or better ways of treatment or new ways to improve the delivery of care. Patients themselves pushed to be treated at home rather than sit for hours on end in a chair or a hospital bed on a drip. I've also been very fortunate to have been able to visit top cancer centres around the world, to see what works and doesn't work. That includes the Memorial Sloan Kettering Cancer Center in New York, the University of Texas MD Anderson Cancer Center and the Mayo Clinic, and I believe the treatment offered at Lifehouse is world standard.

The fact is that as the population of Australia ages, more people will be diagnosed with cancer. When I started in nursing, the average life expectancy for a female was 78 and for a male 76; now it's something like 81–82 years for a man and 83–84 for a woman. People are living into their late 80s and 90s now, and the longer we live, the more likely we are to be diagnosed with a form of cancer. One case in point is that prostate cancer is now the most commonly diagnosed cancer in men. While cancer is also on the increase as a result of environmental factors such as exposure to the sun and smoking- and industry-related lung cancers, and breast cancer and prostate cancers are still prevalent, we are treating an increasing number of patients with new, faster-acting and more effective chemotherapy and targeted drugs. Screening is better too, and you can now expect to receive a bowel cancer screening kit from the federal government as a 50th birthday present. There is also a lot more education and the teaching of precautionary measures in schools and universities, plus there are awareness campaigns, billboards and TV and internet ads. People have also become much more attuned to the fact that if they have a lump or are short of breath or have pain, they should go to see a doctor, and be sent to an oncologist or have a biopsy. Plus we have much better equipment to detect cancers early on, including CT scans, MRIs and PET scans.

Four decades ago, when the treatment of cancer patients was scattered throughout a hospital and not given over to specific cancer care, patients were treated predominantly by general nursing staff, and you could see the shortfalls in that. In those days, we had a very small team of nurses who were cancer-trained. At RPA, the nursing staff went all around the hospital and to the Brown Street outpatients' clinic to treat people with chemotherapy, but we couldn't be there 24/7, so we would have to hand over responsibility to the ward staff. General staff found treating cancer patients both distressing and overwhelming, and even though we tried to educate them, they found it quite daunting because of the new drugs which made people very sick when they took them and often weren't successful.

COVID-19 has added a layer of complexity to nursing that I never had to deal with. This is quite apart from the vast array of changes I saw across my 40 years of nursing. Today, nurses now start their training at university, not in a hospital. They log patient details into a computer and don't have to fill out paper forms. There is day surgery and robotic surgery. Patients don't convalesce for as long. Treatments can be done as an outpatient rather than as an inpatient. Nurses are more process-driven and the feeling I get is that the nurse–patient relationship has changed. Nurses have to do more with less. When people go to the hospital now, they have what needs to be done and then they are discharged and that is that. The nurses and doctors generally don't get to know patients very well.

While advances include having designated hospitals dedicated to cancer patients, the way of thinking and caring for someone with cancer is also different. With cancer, the first thing patients and relatives usually think of is death. As a cancer nurse, compassion and understanding are key, as we get to know many patients extremely well. They could be facing months or years of treatment, so you come to know them not only as a patient but as someone you care about and want to help on that journey. They become friends, as is the case with many of my surviving patients as well as the families of those who have not survived. That broader influence you have over a patient and their welfare continues with their relatives; I continue to maintain contact with several families who have lost loved ones to cancer and I feel very fortunate to call them friends. Some people might be critical of that because it blurs the lines between the professional and the personal, but I think that has made me the nurse I am today.

29

FIRM BELIEVER

While you have to have a little bit of a veneer for your own emotional self-protection, if you can't give something of yourself in the nursing process, I don't think you can do this job properly.

I am a firm believer in the need to look after yourself as well as the patients. Like everyone else, I need time out sometimes, because if you do break down or can't cope, then you are no good to anyone – yourself, the patient, their relatives or your fellow workers. And while you need to get that balance right, it can take a while. I worked out early in my professional life that when we are born, we all embark on some sort of pathway, then we are all going to die, eventually, so I was resolved to these facts of life as I see them. But I also have faith that life doesn't finish here and now. Hopefully, if we lead a good life, we are going to have a better life after this one.

I think having that belief has helped me develop compassionate relationships with patients, plus helped both them and me through some difficult experiences – including watching them take their last breaths. I also believe my faith has given me both strength and understanding. Some might say my religion has been a bit of a crutch, something to lean on when times are tough and yes, I have to agree to a certain extent. But I often think to myself, if I didn't have faith and I didn't have that crutch, what would I have to lean on? For me, faith is the most amazing thing; to have the belief that there is life after death and that you can make a difference before that happens is the most incredible gift.

While I would never force my faith on others, I do think it is the reason I have always tried to be kind and understanding, and I feel it has made me a better person. To be quite honest, I love people and I love being involved in their lives and I would do anything for anyone. I feel enriched by my faith, by receiving communion and communicating with God. I think God has given me a lot of strength and that is why He has put me here, to help and guide people, not only through their treatment but also through their life journey and yes, perhaps their death too. It's an attitude that has enabled me to talk to people who are probably at the lowest point in their lives, when they have just been diagnosed with cancer, or are coming out the other side of treatment, or possibly when both their treatment and their life is at an end. It's a huge honour to walk that path with them.

My faith and my passion have also enabled me to talk to all sorts of people to raise money for charitable organisations, to put on a collar and tie to meet a minister, prime minister or the future king of England, or to have a chat with a homeless person while I'm wearing an apron and serving them a Sunday roast. If you are bright and cheerful and happy with everyone you meet, then that radiates off onto everyone else. But if you are a pessimist and down and depressed, then people don't want to be around you. I'm very fortunate that I've had a fantastic life and I have been able to give and serve and share with so many people. It feels like a gift I've been given.

But I'm not done yet. I still like to go overseas and have already booked my ticket, for when international travel gets back up to speed after COVID-19 that is. I also love to ski and will be hitting the slopes again as soon as we are permitted. Travel and skiing have always been my escape from hospitals and sick people.

After all this time and all my experiences, I am full of respect and admiration for nurses everywhere, especially those of us specialising in cancer nursing. Throughout my career as a cancer nurse, I did what I could to share my experiences with colleagues from across Australia and throughout the world. Knowledge shared is knowledge gained. I have taken interns into my home, including Sam Gibson who became a cancer nurse practitioner in Perth after spending time with me at RPA. Later, after we moved into Lifehouse, we set up a national cancer nurse practitioner (CNP) special interest group within the Cancer Nursing Society of Australia (CNSA), with me as chair, fellow cancer nurse practitioners Jillian Blanchard as deputy chair and Sam as secretary. The special interest group offers support for existing and aspiring cancer nurse practitioners and includes master classes conducted by medical oncologists and other specialists.

I have taught classrooms of nurses from Japan, as well as those medical staff I met in Nepal and Papua New Guinea. I have also been asked to write research papers, from my first in 1983[8] to my last in 2013. I have presented papers at international medical and nursing conferences and I am on the board of several foundations. When Gail O'Brien texted me while I sat at that breakfast table in Perugia, Italy, offering to set up and financially back a scholarship in my name, there were tears of joy in my cappuccino. Over the years there has been little money to help nurses participate in ongoing education, but the Keith Cox Scholarship will now fund overseas study tours and short courses or pay for nurses to attend local or international conferences. The first scholarships were awarded at Lifehouse in 2018 on International Nurses Day, 12 May, which is Florence Nightingale's birthday. Key donors include David Boyer – the brother of my friend and former colleague Michael Boyer – and Julian Hofer, both of whom were patients and have been on the receiving end of the quality cancer nursing care I was able to offer because I was allowed and encouraged to go that step further as a nurse. As Julian told the audience at the scholarship launch, I have been able to connect to the human side of cancer, to treat the person, not only the disease, and this is what has set me apart from many of my peers.

Michael Boyer once said we need more Keiths in this world, and while I can't be cloned – yet – hopefully, with the help of the scholarship, another keen young nurse, possibly from a small country town, will soon be sporting a name badge with the title Cancer Nurse Practitioner proudly etched into it. For a kid from Cullerin, it's a very proud achievement, and one that I couldn't even have imagined when I first walked through Matron's door and sat looking up at those stained-glass windows at Royal Prince Alfred Hospital all those years ago.

ACKNOWLEDGEMENTS

First, I would like to thank Grant Jones, not only for taking on this project but also for putting up with me while writing this book. I would also like to thank my family and friends for their support and encouragement, as well as Kim Burke and her colleague for sage legal advice. I'd especially like to say thank you to those patients and their families who I have mentioned in this book, and I'd also like to thank all the many patients, their families and friends who I came in contact with over 50 years of nursing. A mention must be made of my neighbours, Rebecca and Paddy, who introduced us to copy editor Brianne Collins, who then put us in contact with Pan Macmillan publisher Cate Blake and very helpful editor Belinda Huang. I would also like to thank Tish Lancaster who pulled together *Keith Cox: This Is Your Life*, for my 50th birthday, which was a precursor to this book.

Keith Cox OAM

I would like to offer my heartfelt thanks to my author/journalist mates Matt Condon, Michael Robotham and Charles Cuninghame, who provided advice and guidance from the get-go. Also, Chris O'Brien's daughter Juliette O'Brien, a talented journalist and author who signposted the book-publishing process for us along the way. Chris O'Brien Lifehouse must also be kindly acknowledged for putting us in contact with Luisa Masetto, who transcribed hours and hours of digital recordings, which were often difficult to hear or interpret. She knows both of our voices too well by now. Having coffee with Pan Macmillan publisher Cate Blake was also a godsend, as she quickly understood the motivation behind the book and was so excited about the prospect of publishing Keith's story that she was able to offer a deal memo within hours of our first meeting. I'd also like to thank Belinda Huang and Brianne Collins for cleaning up our often-complicated copy. Last, but certainly not least, I'd like to say thank you to my partner Joan Murphy and my son Louis Jones for their ongoing support and understanding.

Grant Jones

FOUNDATIONS AND SCHOLARSHIPS

I now sit on the Cancer Institute NSW board, and several foundations have been set up after I've helped treat people or have been involved in their lives in some way. It's not only about providing ongoing assistance for them and their family to cope with the death or illness of a loved one, but it also enables friends and families to focus on something positive in life. These foundations have also been created after families have seen shortfalls in funding or levels of care when their relative is being treated.

THE KEITH COX SCHOLARSHIP
After Chris O'Brien died, his wife Gail O'Brien asked if I would accept a scholarship under my name. The Keith Cox Scholarship now funds further education for nurses and allied health practitioners.

donate.mylifehouse.org.au/ways-to-give/other-funds/keith-cox-fund

LIFEHOUSE FOUNDATION
I am a member of the foundation committee, the team which helps raise awareness of the good work done at Lifehouse. Donations to Lifehouse go to research and the improvement of patient care and also to support a nurse specialist in an area of need.

donate.mylifehouse.org.au/ways-to-give/one-off-donation

THE COOPER RICE-BRADING FOUNDATION
Sarcoma is one of the deadliest forms of cancer in children and young adults, and mortality rates have seen no improvement in almost 40 years. This foundation aims to provide the long-term funding required to find a cure for sarcoma, to increase awareness, promote early diagnosis and provide support and guidance to patients and families throughout treatment and beyond.

www.crbf.org.au

THE CANCER INSTITUTE NSW
Chaired by former NSW Premier Morris Iemma, the institute works with stakeholders to reduce the impact of cancer on our community through a range of programs and initiatives. Key partners include the NSW and federal governments, local and state health services and the cancer research community, including GPs and clinical practice nurses, as well as Indigenous-controlled community health organisations and multicultural health services.

www.cancer.nsw.gov.au

THE DANIEL FERGUSON FOUNDATION

Daniel has Limb Girdle Muscular Dystrophy (Type R1) and was diagnosed with this degenerative muscular disorder at the age of 13. I met his father Rick on a Battlefields tour with the Order of Australia Association. Rick's wife Therese was also a nurse, and we share the same faith and have since become firm friends. They watch on as Daniel, now 37, struggles with day-to-day life. While I know all there is to know about cancer, muscular dystrophy is my new challenge.

www.dffoundation.com.au

THE BIAGGIO SIGNORELLI FOUNDATION

Biaggio Signorelli's dying wish was to help others with meso-thelioma, so his son Paul and his two daughters, Anna and Nina, established the Biaggio Signorelli Foundation. Paul asked me to join the board in 2009, and its first chairman was former NSW Premier Morris Iemma, who I know well. The foundation has since raised millions, creating awareness about the disease and helping those who have it.

biaggiosignorelli.org.au

I am very fortunate in life that I have met such incredible people and that they have asked me to contribute to these causes.

CITATIONS

1. Cox K.M., Stuart-Harris R., Abdini G., Grygiel J., Raghavan D. 'The management of cytotoxic drug extravasation: Guidelines drawn up by a working party for the Clinical Oncological Society of Australia.' *The Medical Journal of Australia*, 148, 185–189 (1988).
2. Cox K.M., Hatch M., Delany J., Kerr L., Lawrence K., Fursdon J., Walton F. 'A Pilot Study of High Dose Cisplatin Chemotherapy Given in an Outpatient Setting.' Presented at the 10th International Conference on Cancer Nursing, Jerusalem, Israel (September 1998).
3. Findlay M., Simes J., Cox K.M., Carmichael K., Chey T., McNeil E., Raghavan D. 'A randomised crossover trial of anti-emetic therapy for platinum-based chemotherapy improved control with intensive multiagent regime.' *European Journal of Cancer*, Vol. 29A, No. 3, 309–315 (1993).

4. Cox K., Goel S., O'Connell R., Boyer M., Beale P., Simes J., Stockler M. 'Randomized cross-over trial comparing inpatient and outpatient administration of high-dose Cisplatin.' *Internal Medicine Journal*, Vol. 41, 172–178 (2010).

5. Cox K.M., Visintin L., Kovac S., Childs A., Kelleher H., Murray B., White G., Storey D., Findlay M. 'Establishing a program for continuous ambulatory infusion chemotherapy.' *Journal of Medicine*, Vol. 27, No. 6, 680–684 (December 1997).

6. Clark K., Cox K.M., Allsopp K., Boyer M. 'A longitudinal study to document the benefits and risks associated with the subcutaneous placement of a peritoneal Port-A-Cath to treat refractory malignant ascites: Results from the first 12 months.' Presented at the Palliative Care Conference, Melbourne (August 2007).

7. Coupe N., Cox K., Clarke K., Boyer M., Stockler M. 'Outcomes of permanent peritoneal ports for the management of recurrent malignant ascites.' *Journal of Palliative Medicine*, Vol. 16, No. 8 (2013).

8. Cox K.M. 'Antiemetic trial for use with Cisplatin.' *Oncology Nursing Forum*, Vol. 10, 4:69 (1983).